Clinical Film Viewing Series

AF085581

CARDIOVASCULAR SYSTEM

Clinical Film Viewing Series

Series Editor: Paul R. Goddard BSc, MBBS, MD, DMRD, FRCR

CARDIOVASCULAR SYSTEM

George G. Hartnell BSc(Hons), MBChB, MRCP, FRCR
Consultant in Radiodiagnosis, Bristol Royal Infirmary and
Bristol Royal Hospital for Sick Children

Honorary Senior Lecturer in Diagnostic Radiology,
Royal Postgraduate Medical School, Hammersmith Hospital

with a Foreword by

Professor E. R. Davies, CBE Professor of
Radiodiagnosis, University of Bristol

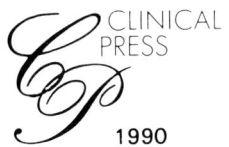

1990

© **Clinical Press Limited.** 1990

All Rights Reserved. No part of this publication may be reproduced, stored in a retrieval system, or transmitted in any form or by any means, electronic, mechanical, photocopying, recording or otherwise, without the prior permission of the Copyright owner.

Published by:
Clinical Press Limited
Registered Office, Redland Green Farm,
Redland Green, Redland, Bristol, BS6 7HF

British Library Cataloguing in Publication Data
Hartnell, George G.
  Cardiovascular system.
  1.   Man. Cardiovascular system. Diagnosis
  I.   Title   II. Series
  616.1'075

ISBN 1-85457-012-9

Typeset by:
Severntype Repro Services Ltd,
Kingswood, Wotton-under-Edge, GL12 8RL

Printed in Great Britain by:
Manor Printing Services (Wotton) Ltd,
The Abbey Business Park, Charfield Road,
Kingswood, Wotton-under-Edge, GL12 8RL

Contents

Foreword	vii
Series Editor's Foreword	viii
Introduction	ix
Acknowledgements	x
Eighty Diagnostic Exercises	1
Index	163

Foreword

by **Professor E. R. Davies** CBE

The archetype of British medical teaching is the illustrated case. It has been the backbone of all the ward rounds and radiological tutorials that we have ever attended. As the body of radiological knowledge increased, systematic collection of data in comprehensive textbooks became necessary and so did the need for systematic lecture programmes. The received wisdom from these sources deserved to be validated and enlarged by serious research and the robust health of our journals attests the quality of such research.

The student of radiology—whatever his seniority or professional persuasion—thus has unrivalled resources of data. And yet the day-to-day commerce of clinical radiology trades in the art of applying this information to specific case problems. This art can only be acquired by supervised practice and experience. The importance of acquiring it is emphasised in the structure of the final FRCR Examination which contains a film reporting component carrying considerable weight. Postgraduate examinations in medicine and surgery and other clinical subjects now also have a similar film viewing section.

Dr George Hartnell, an experienced and enthusiastic teacher, has the ideal attributes for driving home the importance of eliciting signs meticulously, of presenting the problem concisely, and of discussing the contribution of established relevant data. On these lines he has written an invaluable learning book derived from his own special interests in Diagnostic Radiology. All good teaching of this kind is strengthened by an unequivocal expression of a personal viewpoint where some controversy may exist. Dr Hartnell's book is a vital stone in the mosaic of this Clinical Film Viewing Series.

E. Rhys Davies
Professor of Radiodiagnosis
University of Bristol

Series Editor's Foreword

Many of the postgraduate examinations now include radiographic interpretation which may be presented as a slide show or as a film-viewing session. In addition, radiographs and other imaging modalities are used ubiquitously in the 'viva' section of most major postgraduate examinations including those of the American Boards and of professional societies and universities world wide.

In a typical examination situation candidates are asked to view a film but are provided with minimal clinical information. They are then asked to give a written or oral report together with a sensible list of possible differential diagnoses.

It is the intention of this series of books on *Clinical Film Viewing* to assist the candidates in preparing themselves for this process. Each book examines a particular system or technique and promotes the reader's own self-questioning about the films presented.

The *Clinical Film Viewing Series* provides a unique opportunity for self-assessment and learning in all the modern modalities of diagnostic imaging.

Paul R. Goddard

Introduction

By its nature the cardiovascular system extends throughout the body and involves all of the different organ systems. For the purposes of this book the disorders of the cardiovascular system which are illustrated will be confined to diseases of the heart and diseases specifically of the blood vessels themselves, rather than of the organs they supply.

This book is aimed at candidates for postgraduate examinations in all specialties and especially those doctors with some training in cardiovascular disease who need to assess their knowledge of the subject. The book is particularly applicable to candidates for postgraduate examinations in radiology.

The cases which are illustrated reflect the types of case which may be presented in radiographic form in postgraduate medical examinations. Some of these conditions are common but have a number of different manifestations, others are rare but have characteristic appearances which should be well known. A number of cases deliberately deal with different aspects of the same condition. This reflects in part the numerical importance of these conditions in clinical practice and examinations and in part the frequency with which the diagnoses are missed or inappropriate investigations are carried out. This applies especially to the interpretation of the chest radiograph, which is usually the initial radiological examination in patients with cardiovascular disease. It provides diagnostic and functional information which is all too often ignored or misinterpreted.

Particular attention is paid to the role of newer imaging and interventional techniques with which examination candidates should be familiar, even if they have little personal experience of these techniques. There is no doubt that these techniques will become even more widely available and trainees should be aware of them and be able to discuss their applications. Some techniques are difficult to illustrate and are more useful for providing functional rather than anatomical information which makes reporting on a single image impossible. For this reason some investigations, in particular isotope studies, are only sparsely represented.

This book should be used as a self-assessment aid in film interpretation as well as providing a guide to the discussion which may follow the interpretation of radiographic data in examinations. However, books can never be a substitute for viewing a very large number of radiographs and reporting on them, preferably under stressful examination-like conditions.

The cases illustrated are divided into two sections. The first ten cases should be reported as one would report in an examination. Each case is followed by a specimen report which records the important abnormal features and the relevant normal features shown. Only relevant clinical data are given with each case. Following the specimen report is a discussion which deals with those topics which may be raised in a typical examination. In the remaining seventy cases specific questions are asked. The answers to specific questions on diagnosis or technique are identified by Capital Letters Thus.

Acknowledgements

Thanks are due to the following people for their assistance in the preparation of this book:

The Medical Illustration Department, Bristol Royal Infirmary, for making most of the illustrations and managing to reproduce even the most difficult radiographs.

Paul Goddard and Clinical Press for providing the stimulus to start this project.

E. Merck for encouragement and support from a very early stage.

Sarah Smith for correcting my grammatical and spelling errors.

Professor David Allison and Professor Anne Hemingway for their help and encouragement over the years and for permission to reproduce *Figs* 22, 73 and 79 (Professor Allison) and *Fig.* 30 (Professor Hemingway).

CARDIOVASCULAR SYSTEM

Case 1

Report on this chest radiograph of an elderly female patient admitted with severe chest pain and hypotension.

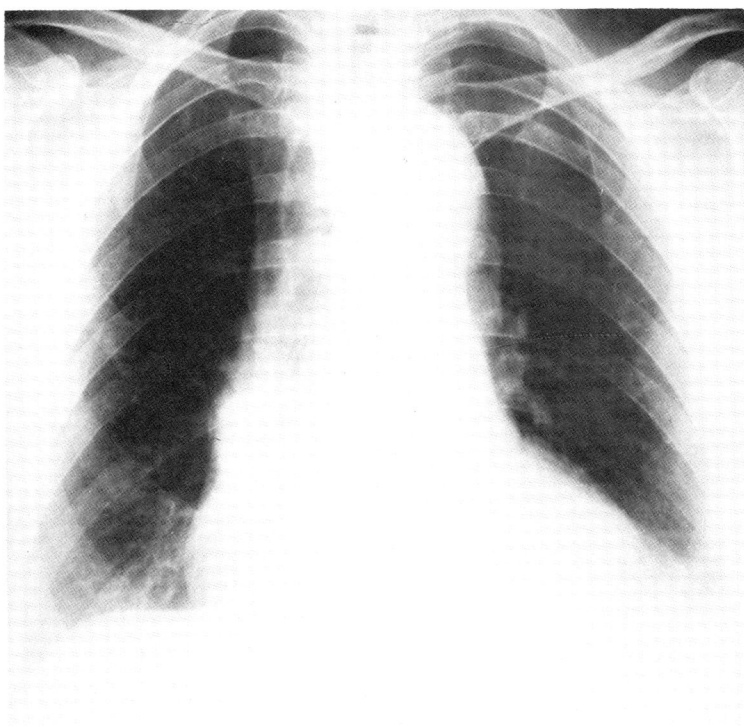

Figure 1a

Specimen Report

'The heart is enlarged and there is widening of the aortic arch with deviation of the trachea to the right. There is a left pleural effusion but the rest of the lung fields are clear. In this patient the radiological features suggest dissection of the aorta and further investigation by echocardiography and dynamic enhanced CT are suggested. The large cardiac outline suggests that the patient may have been hypertensive or that there is a haemopericardium.'

This patient had indeed been hypertensive for many years and the diagnosis of aortic dissection was confirmed by computed tomography (CT, *Fig.* 1 *b*) which clearly showed a dissection flap in the descending aorta and a less clear flap in the ascending aorta (DeBakey Type 1 dissection). Echocardiography may show the flap in the aorta and is also necessary to demonstrate aortic regurgitation and haemopericardium. Aortography is seldom necessary to demonstrate the anatomy and is less sensitive than dynamic CT for making the diagnosis. The reason for this can be seen in *Fig.* 1 *b*. The false lumen is often thin and curves around the true lumen, making it impossible to separate the two on most conventional angiographic projections. The sectional nature of CT and the better contrast resolution of CT overcomes this problem very well.

These patients are in an extremely precarious situation and investigation is required as a matter of considerable urgency. If the diagnosis is suspected from the chest radiograph this information must be transmitted quickly to the clinicians dealing with the patient.

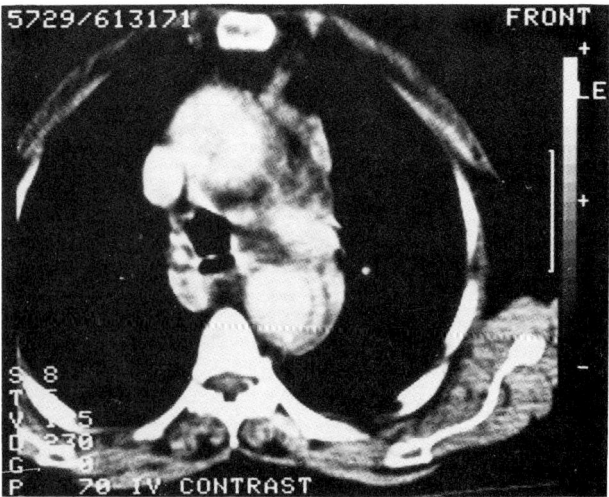

Figure 1 *b*

CARDIOVASCULAR SYSTEM

Case 2

This patient was referred to clinic following the discovery of a murmur. Report on this chest radiograph. What further investigation would you advise?

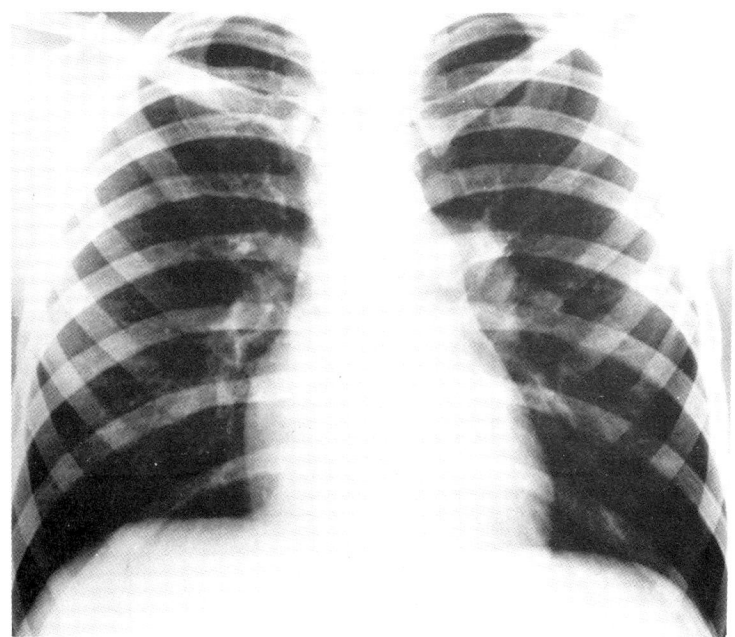

Figure 2a

Specimen Report

'The heart is not enlarged but there is prominence of the main pulmonary artery and the proximal left pulmonary artery. The proximal right and the peripheral pulmonary arteries are of normal size. The lung fields are normal. The appearances suggest pulmonary valve stenosis. Echocardiography with Doppler is advised to confirm this and to assess the severity of the gradient.'

This is a characteristic appearance. The absence of cardiac enlargement is an important negative feature to mention in this case, although negative features which are not relevant should not be placed in such a prominent position when being discussed. Cardiomegaly would indicate that there is more severe heart disease, such as mitral valve disease or an ASD, complicated by pulmonary hypertension. Prominence of the main and left pulmonary artery is a not uncommon finding in young women, but this patient appears to be male. A similar appearance can be produced by pectus excavatum but there are no other features of this on this radiograph.

Echocardiography with continuous-wave Doppler can confirm the diagnosis in the majority of patients and is often the only investigation required. If a severe gradient is found this can be confirmed at cardiac catheterization, which can be combined with balloon pulmonary valvoplasty. *Fig.* 2*b* shows a thickened but well-formed, doming stenotic valve of the type which is suitable for valvoplasty.

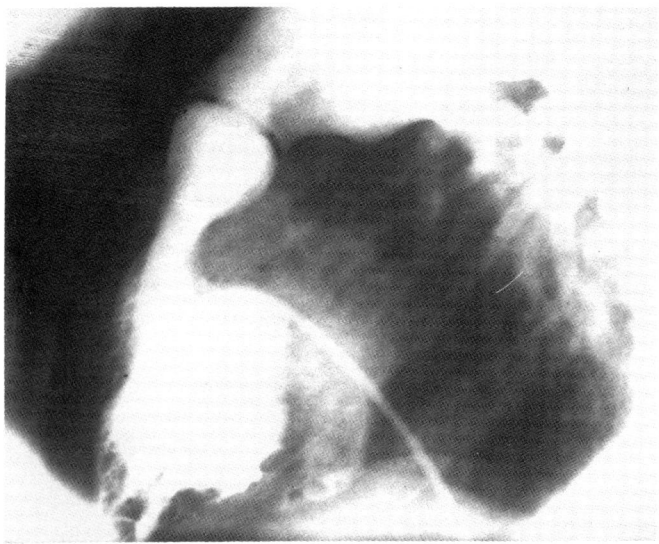

Figure 2*b*

Case 3

Report on this chest radiograph. What further investigations would you advise to assess the importance of your findings?

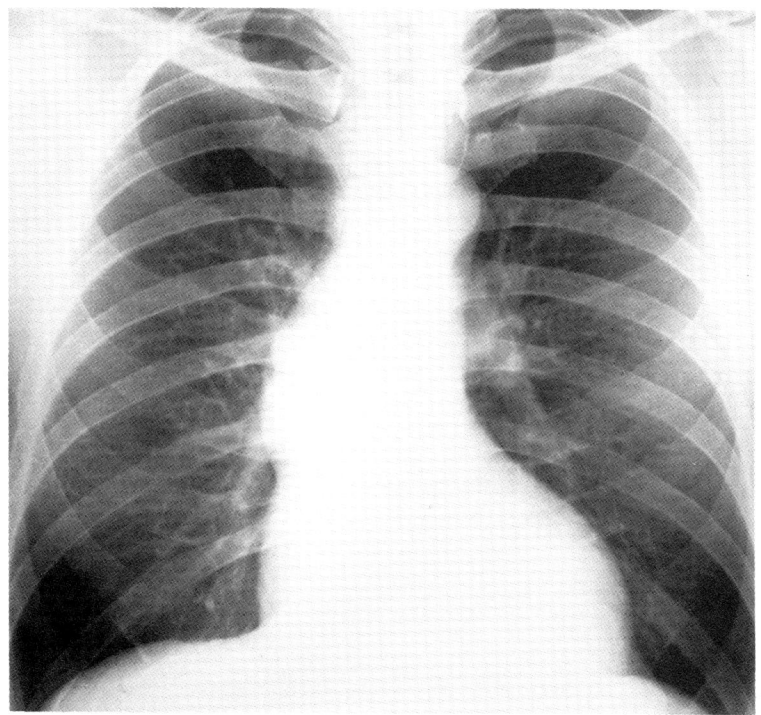

Figure 3a

Specimen Report

'The heart size is normal but there is marked prominence of the ascending aorta. The aortic arch and descending aorta are not dilated. The pulmonary arteries are not dilated and the lungs appear normal. These features are suggestive of aortic valve disease. In view of the degree of aortic dilatation in the absence of cardiac enlargement the dominant lesion is more likely to be aortic stenosis than regurgitation.'

A lateral view confirms that the aortic valve is calcified (*Fig. 3b*). The next useful investigation is echocardiography to assess left ventricular function, to confirm the diagnosis of calcific aortic stenosis and to evaluate the state of the other cardiac valves, in particular the mitral valve. Continuous-wave Doppler will accurately predict the degree of stenosis and pulsed or colour-flow Doppler will assess the degree of aortic regurgitation. Cardiac catheterization is usually only necessary if the coronary arteries need to be shown, particularly in patients with chest pain, prior to valve replacement.

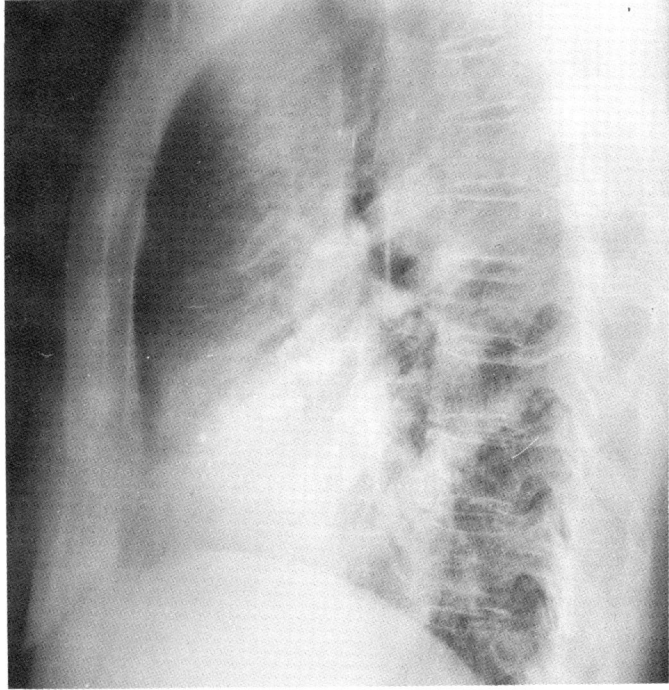

Figure 3b

CARDIOVASCULAR SYSTEM

Case 4

Write a report on this chest radiograph taken of a 55-year-old gentleman.

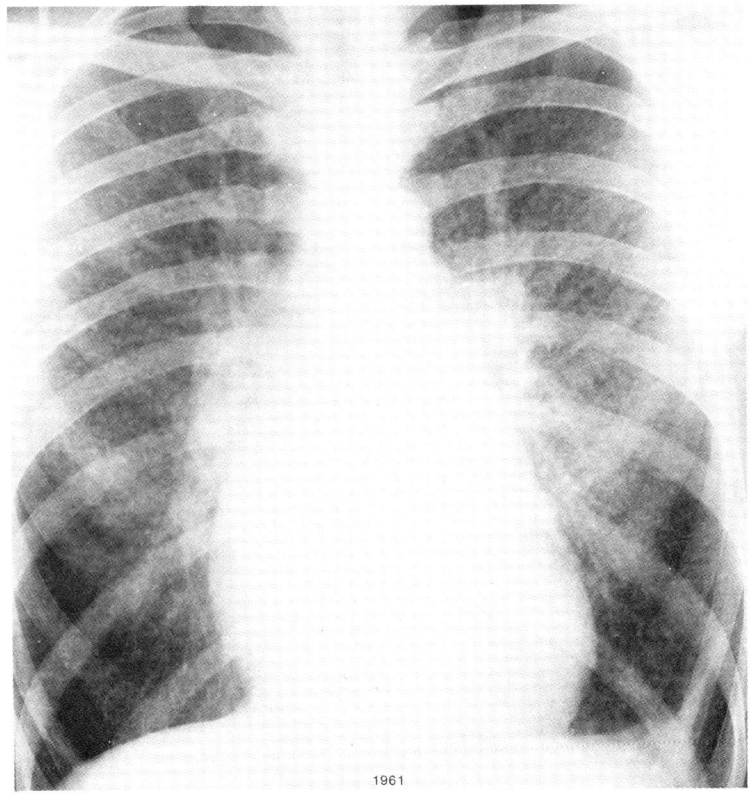

Figure 4a

Specimen Report

'The heart size is at the upper limit of normal and there is enlargement of the left atrium (as shown by a prominent left atrial appendage and a double right heart border). The main pulmonary artery is large and there is a very large number of fine punctate, medium density shadows throughout both lung fields, especially in the mid-zones. There is no evidence of surgery. These are the features of chronic mitral valve disease, predominantly stenosis, with pulmonary hypertension and pulmonary haemosiderosis. An echocardiogram is advised to confirm the diagnosis and to assess the severity of the stenosis.'

The absence of any signs of surgery is an important negative feature. The features of mitral stenosis are clear and the presence of haemosiderosis indicates that significant stenosis has been present for a long time.

Although a lateral chest radiograph is usually taken this adds little further important information. The next useful investigation should be an echocardiogram, including Doppler. Echocardiography will give information on left atrial size and the presence of atrial thrombus, left ventricular function, mitral calcification and valve disease elsewhere. Pulsed and continuous-wave Doppler will quantify the degree of mitral regurgitation and give a good estimate of mitral valve area. *Fig.* 4*b* is a continuous wave Doppler trace from another patient showing a prolonged pressure half-time (half-time = 262 ms indicating a mitral valve area of 0·84 cm^2).

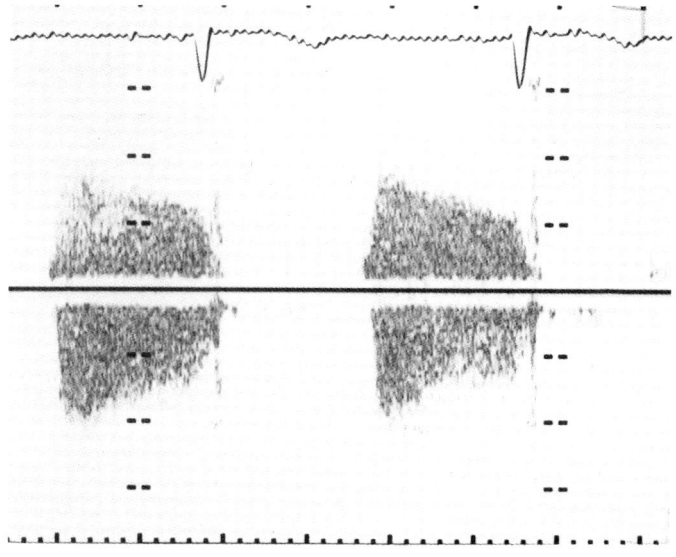

Figure 4*b*

CARDIOVASCULAR SYSTEM

Case 5

Write a report on this chest radiograph of a 1-year-old child. The child was once cyanosed but was not cyanosed at the time of this examination.

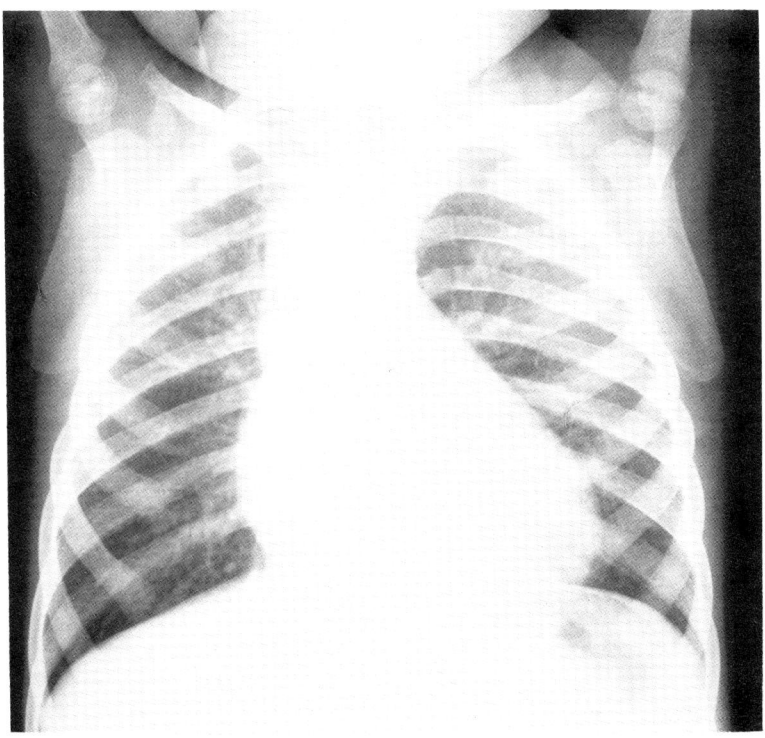

Figure 5

Specimen Report

'There is a straight left heart border with small proximal pulmonary arteries and poor peripheral pulmonary arteries. There is a well-defined shadow to the right of the superior mediastinum and there is malalignment of the right 5th rib as it passes the lateral chest wall. The heart is not enlarged. The features are those of a patient who has had a Blalock type shunt for cyanotic congenital heart disease, such as Fallot's tetralogy or pulmonary atresia.'

There may also be a suggestion of an elevated cardiac apex but, as is usually the case at this age, this is a rather subtle change of dubious diagnostic value unless there are other features to accompany it.

The key to this film is the shadow extending down from just below the right clavicle to the level of the right pulmonary artery with the associated malalignment of the right 5th rib. The shadow is the Blalock shunt (of which there are several types). The minor malalignment of the 5th rib indicates the site of a lateral thoracotomy; not all thoracotomies cause the characteristic rib irregularity which makes the diagnosis easier to identify. Even if the shunt is difficult to see, evidence of a right lateral thoracotomy in a patient with congenital heart disease is strong evidence of a shunt procedure of some sort. Although this information is usually available in clinical practice it may not be volunteered in examinations. In examinations, however, the information about the presence or absence of cyanosis should be given as this is critical to the differential diagnosis. On the left other procedures can be performed through a lateral thoracotomy (i.e. coarctation repair, ductus ligation) but again evidence of a thoracotomy should prompt a search for evidence of a shunt. The presence of a shunt, small proximal pulmonary arteries, oligaemia and right ventricular hypertrophy (elevated cardiac apex) are features of both Fallot's tetralogy and pulmonary atresia. Shunts are also found in patients with other types of right heart obstruction such as tricuspid atresia.

CARDIOVASCULAR SYSTEM

Case 6

Report on this chest radiograph of a patient with a cardiac murmur.

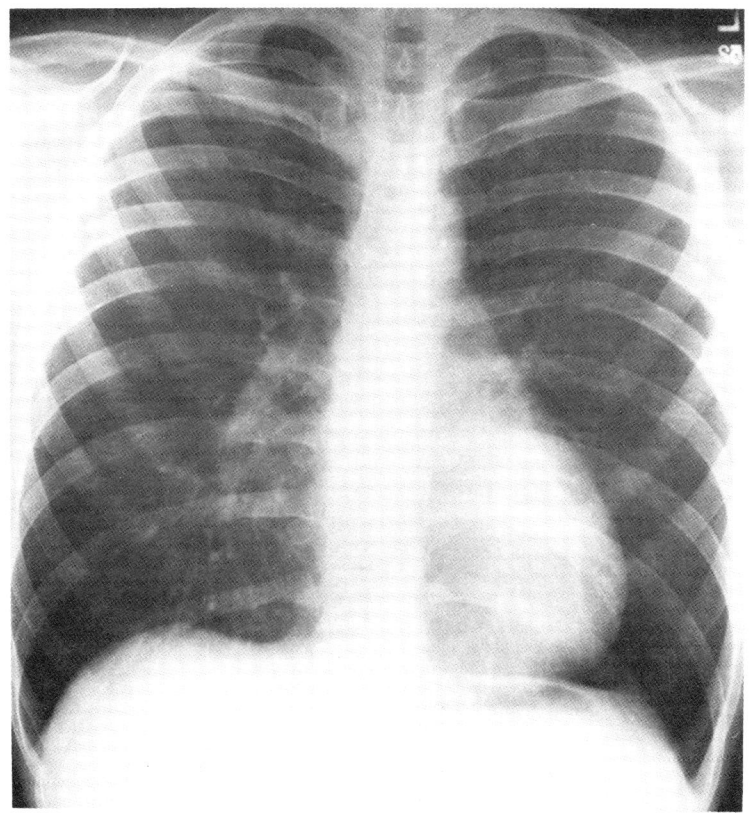

Figure 6a

Specimen Report

'The heart is displaced to the left but is not enlarged. The posterior portions of the ribs are abnormally horizontal and the anterior portions of the ribs are orientated more vertically than is normal. There is an area of increased shadowing in the right lower zone medially. These are the features of pectus excavatum.'

There is a temptation in examinations, and in practice, to say more about straightforward radiographs than is necessary. In this case the radiographic features are diagnostic and no further comment or investigation is required. Although this patient had a lateral chest radiograph (*Fig. 6b*), which confirmed the diagnosis, this should not be suggested as a confirmatory examination. If confirmation is required, examining the patient's chest will do this and avoid unnecessary expense and radiation exposure. In this case the policy of the outpatient clinic was to request a PA and lateral chest radiograph on all new patients.

Examination technique: Do not ask for unnecessary investigations because they are commonly requested. Unnecessary examinations cost money and expose the population to unnecessary radiation, and a small risk of developing malignancies in later life. It is important that anyone requesting a radiographic examination understands this and seriously considers what the benefit to the patient of any investigation will be, compared to the potential risks, and whether the same information could be obtained by a safer method, such as clinical examination.

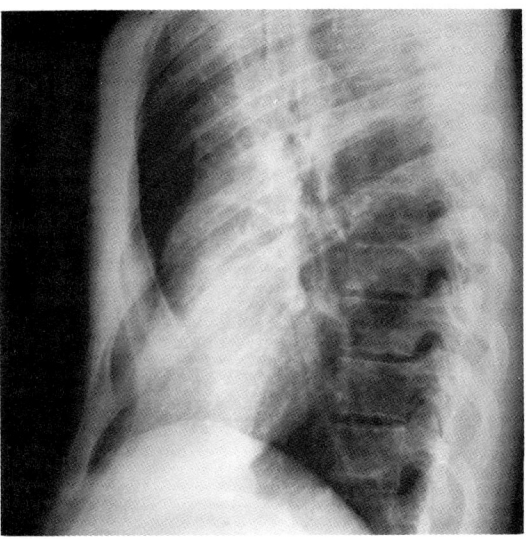

Figure 6b

Case 7

Report on this chest radiograph of a child born 12 hours earlier. Following a normal pregnancy and delivery the child rapidly became ill with **tachypnoea, cyanosis** and **acidosis**.

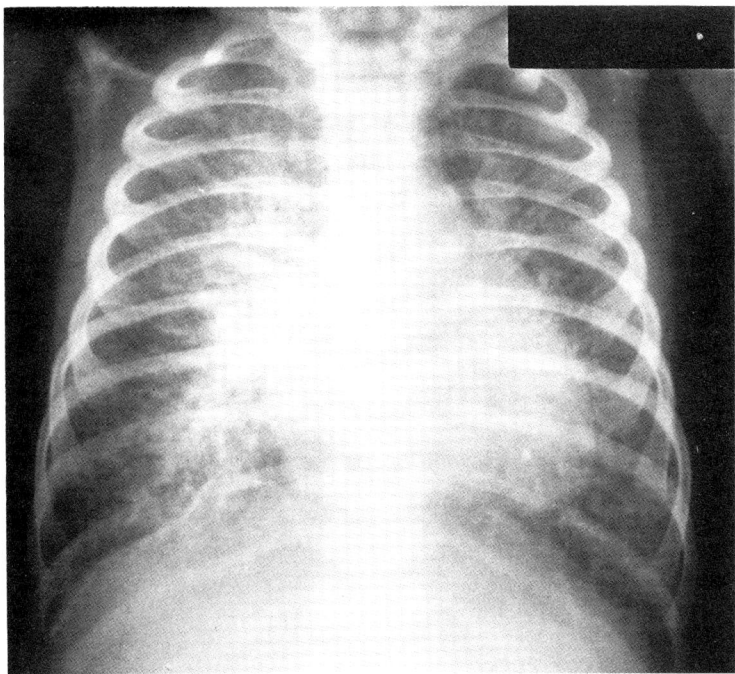

Figure 7a

Specimen Report

'The heart size is normal but there is an increase in pulmonary vascular markings with extensive alveolar shadowing in both lung fields. The features suggest pulmonary venous congestion and pulmonary oedema. In a patient of this age the differential diagnosis includes hypoplastic left heart syndrome, obstructed total anomalous pulmonary venous drainage and pulmonary lymphangiectasia. Echocardiography is advised to demonstrate the cardiac anatomy and the pulmonary venous drainage.'

There are other causes of this radiographic appearance but not all of these are appropriate in the clinical setting. The other possibilities which are less likely include transient respiratory distress of the newborn, amniotic fluid aspiration, hypervolaemia, hyperviscosity, intracranial haemorrhage (all of which are less severe clinically and tend to improve over the 24–48 hours following delivery), severe coarctation or asphyxiated myocardium (both usually associated with significant cardiomegaly), pulmonary angiomatosis (very rare). The comment on normal heart size is relevant to the differential diagnosis and therefore appears in the first sentence of the report. If it is not relevant it should be relegated to a less prominent position. In this case the diagnosis of obstructed (infradiaphragmatic) total anomalous pulmonary venous drainage was confirmed by angiography (*Fig.* 7*b*).

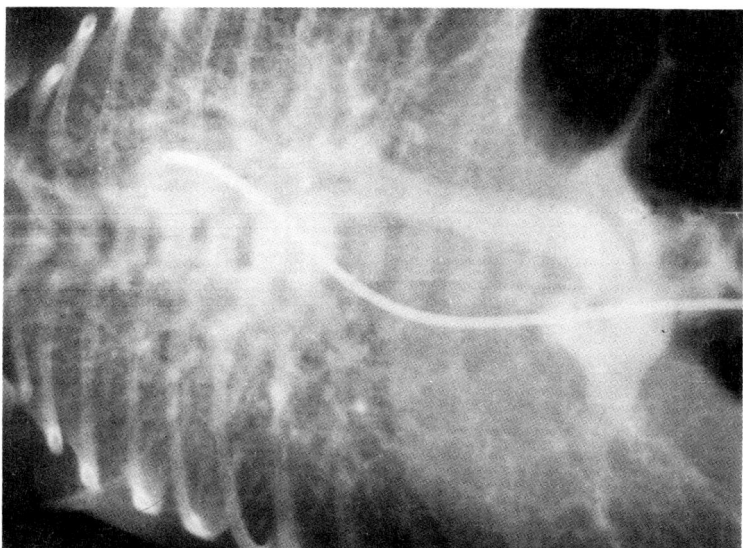

Figure 7*b*

Case 8

Report on this chest radiograph of a 50-year-old patient admitted as an emergency with severe chest pain, dyspnoea and confusion.

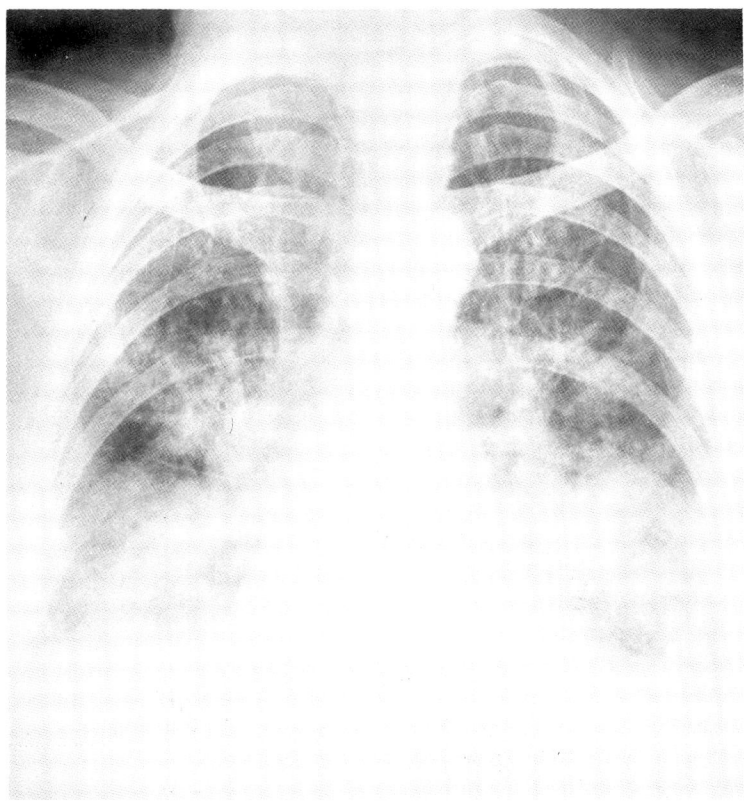

Figure 8

Specimen Report

'There is extensive bilateral alveolar shadowing, particularly in the lower zones, bilateral small pleural effusions and fluid in the horizontal fissure. The upper lobe pulmonary veins are prominent and the heart size is at the upper limit of normal. The features are those of pulmonary oedema which could be due to a number of causes of which myocardial infarction is probably the most likely.'

In this case the presence of pulmonary venous distension is important in differentiating pulmonary oedema from the other causes of extensive alveolar shadowing which could mimic this appearance (including the broad categories of pulmonary infection, pulmonary haemorrhage, pulmonary eosinophilia, alveolar proteinosis). Pulmonary venous distension also helps to exclude the causes of pulmonary oedema in which the pulmonary venous pressure is normal (i.e. adult respiratory distress syndrome, drowning, drug overdose). Clearly many of these are also excluded by the history.

The differential diagnosis now lies between the cardiogenic causes of pulmonary oedema and the non-cardiogenic causes of pulmonary oedema which also cause an increase in pulmonary venous pressure. In the clinical context the suggestion of myocardial infarction (possibly complicated by mitral valve dysfunction or an infarct ventricular septal defect) is a reasonable suggestion. However, other causes must not be excluded on the radiographic appearances. The alternative diagnoses include acute or chronic renal failure and the many other causes of fluid overload. In this particular case the patient had chronic renal failure with fluid overload and uraemic pericarditis, which was the cause of his chest pain.

Case 9

This patient had a myocardial infarction four months previously. Immediately prior to his discharge from hospital at that time his chest radiograph was normal. Report on his current chest radiograph.

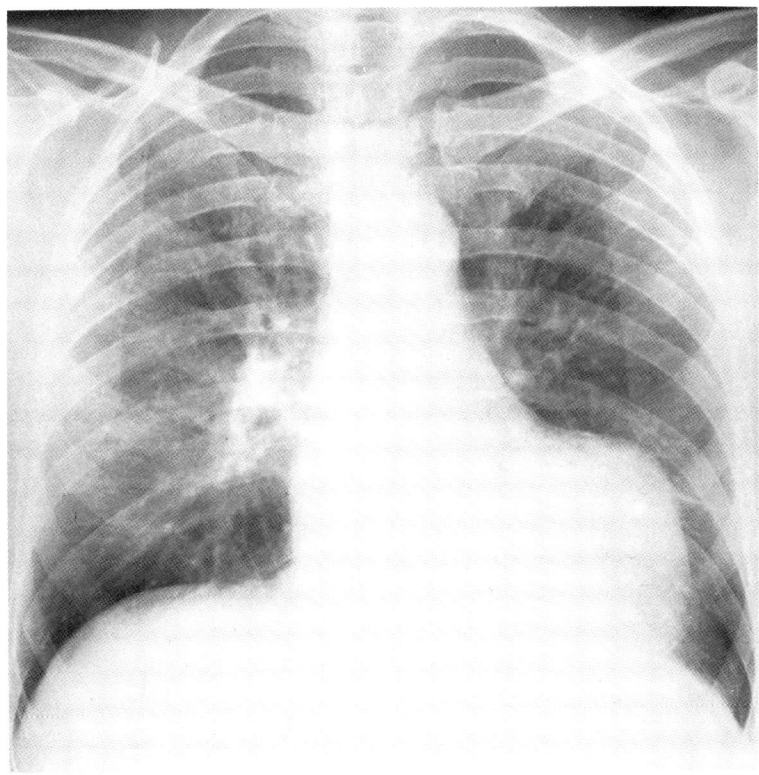

Figure 9a

Specimen Report

'The heart is enlarged and has an abnormal configuration with a prominent angled left heart border. The pulmonary vessels in the upper zones are prominent. The appearances suggest the development of a left ventricular aneurysm and a degree of pulmonary venous congestion. Further investigation by isotope ventriculography to confirm this is suggested.'

This report is short because there are only two significant abnormalities, one of which is very clear and characteristic. The cardiac outline is typical of a left ventricular aneurysm (although a similar appearance can rarely occur with pericardial fat pads or tumours) and the history is consistent with this diagnosis. Isotope ventriculography is the easiest non-invasive method for confirming this diagnosis. Although echocardiography can also show left ventricular aneurysms these patients with ischaemic heart disease are often poor subjects for echocardiographic examinations. MRI and, to a lesser extent, CT can also demonstrate left ventricular aneurysms.

Prior to definitive surgical treatment cardiac catheterization is required to confirm the diagnosis and to demonstrate the coronary artery anatomy. This usually shows total occlusion of the offending artery, usually the left anterior descending artery (as shown in *Fig. 9b*) with poor collateral supply distal to the obstruction. In cases where the aneurysm has been present for a long time there may be calcification in the wall of the aneurysm (as indicated in *Fig. 9b*).

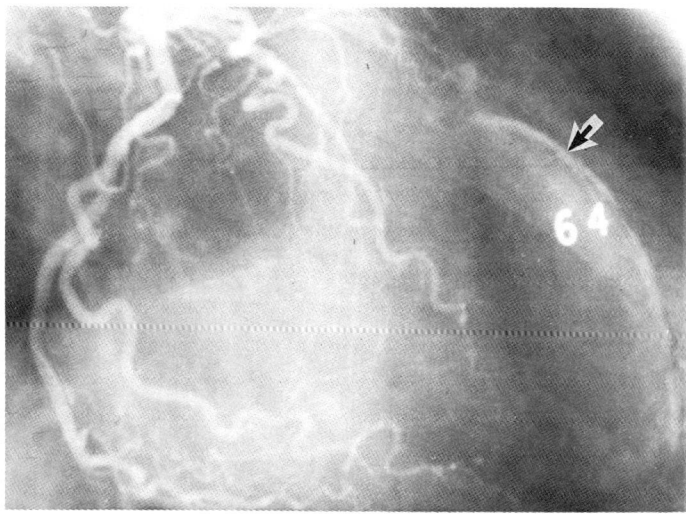

Figure 9b

Case 10

Report on this chest radiograph from a young adult patient. What might the history on the request form be?

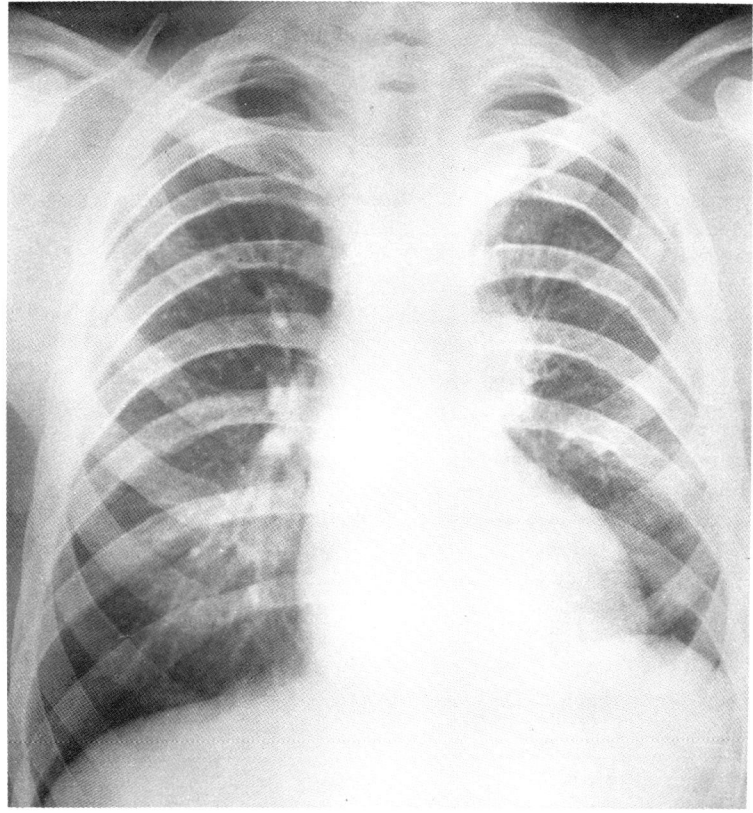

Figure 10

Specimen Report

'There is an unusually high aortic arch which extends up to the level of the left clavicle. There is also a bulge in the descending aorta at the level of the left hilum. There is bilateral rib notching but no other rib abnormality, the heart is not enlarged and there is no evidence of heart failure. This suggests that there is significant coarctation of the aorta and further investigation is advised.' In this case the type of further investigation depends on the local availability of various techniques.

The likely history in this case is that the patient presented with hypertension and a systolic murmur. Coarctation diagnosed in childhood is usually treated surgically in childhood, hence the comment about the absence of any other rib abnormalities which might indicate previous surgery.

The elongated high aortic arch with bilateral rib notching, although the notching is not very marked, makes the diagnosis of coarctation almost certain. There are many other causes of bilateral rib notching but these are less common and none are associated with this type of aortic configuration. The presence of rib notching indicates that there is a significant gradient across the coarctation and this should be confirmed clinically. The method of demonstrating the coarctation prior to surgery depends on the availability of different imaging methods and the willingness of the surgeon to accept the results obtained. In general the least invasive method for imaging the coarctation should be used. If available this would be MRI, possibly augmented by Doppler to assess the gradient across the coarctation. In adults echocardiography is less satisfactory in the demonstration of coarctation, although it is very useful in young children. Intravenous digital subtraction angiography (i.v. DSA) is a satisfactory alternative but if this is not available conventional angiography may be required.

There is an increased incidence of aortic valve disease in these patients (up to 85 per cent have a bicuspid aortic valve) and there is usually hypertension proximal to the coarctation, hence the comments on the normal heart size and absence of evidence of heart failure are relevant to the report.

Case 11

This is an arch aortogram performed on a 28-year-old woman. How was it performed? What does it show? What are the possible causes of this appearance?

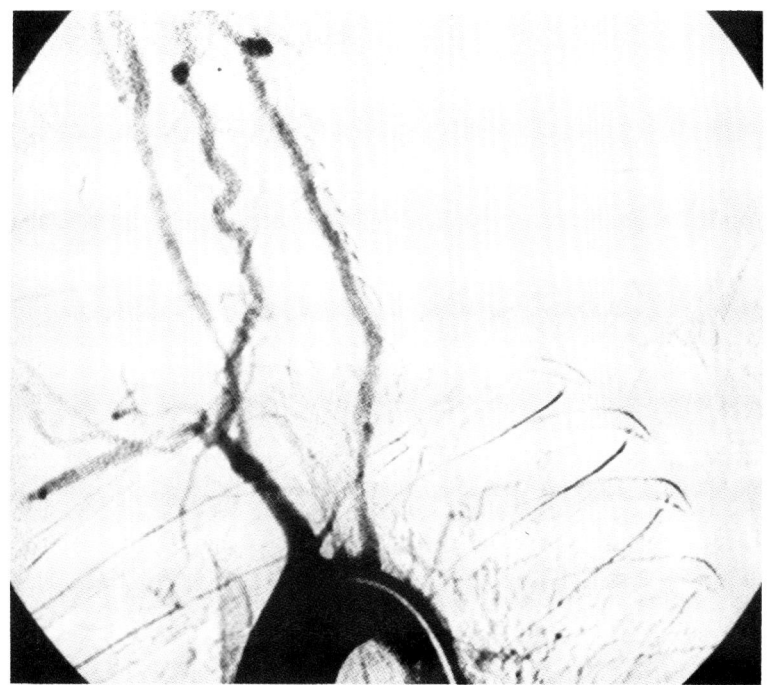

Figure 11

The arch aortogram has been taken in the Left Anterior Oblique projection using Intra-arterial Digital Subtraction Angiography (i.a. DSA). The left vertebral artery is patent but the left subclavian artery beyond this is occluded. The left common carotid artery is completely occluded (the stump is just visible). The right common carotid artery is narrowed proximally and the right subclavian artery is also small. Both the vertebral arteries are large.

In a patient of this age there are only a few possible differential diagnoses. This pattern of widespread proximal arterial stenosis and occlusion is typical of Takayasu's disease, which most commonly affects young Oriental women. Similar appearances occur in the occlusive form of arterial disease sometimes seen in Behçet's disease, and this was the diagnosis in this patient. A similar appearance could be produced by extensive atherosclerosis but this would be very unlikely in a female patient of this age.

Takayasu's disease can affect both the systemic and pulmonary arteries. It produces a progressive narrowing of arteries leading to occlusion and hypertrophy of collateral vessels, provided that these are not also involved in the disease process. The effects of the disease depend on the arteries involved. Arterial calcification may be visible on plain radiographs.

Behçet's disease most commonly affects the venous parts of the circulation, typically causing recurrent thrombophlebitis. In the minority in whom the arteries are involved the disease can be manifest as either an occlusive process (as in this case) or it can produce arterial dilatation with aneurysm formation, which can lead to rupture. Any artery can be involved but there is usually involvement of the aorta and the other proximal major vessels.

CARDIOVASCULAR SYSTEM

Case 12

What is this procedure and what condition is it being used to treat? What are the indications for this procedure and what are the potential complications? What other conditions are suitable for this type of treatment?

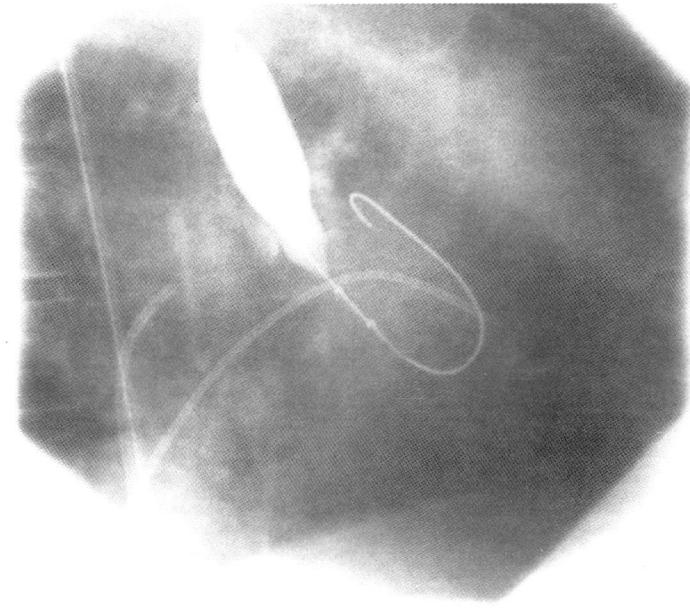

Figure 12*a*

This is a Percutaneous Balloon Valvoplasty which in this case is being used to treat Calcific Aortic Stenosis (note the ring of valve calcification surrounding the balloon). Balloon aortic valvoplasty can be performed from either an arterial approach, as shown in *Fig.* 12*a*, or a transeptal venous approach, as shown in *Fig.* 12*b*. This is a palliative procedure which is indicated for the treatment of aortic stenosis in patients who are unsuitable for aortic valve replacement. This may be due to Advanced Age, Very Poor Left Ventricular Function, Extensive Inoperable Coronary Artery Disease, Severe Non-Cardiac Disease (i.e. respiratory, renal or malignant disease). As techniques improve the indications are becoming wider and now also includes Refusal of Surgery by the patient.

Potential complications include systemic embolization, excessive aortic regurgitation, haemorrhage from the puncture site, haemopericardium, femoral arteriovenous fistula, femoral artery occlusion and arrhythmias. In spite of this rather daunting list of complications the procedure is now accepted as a useful procedure, in a previously untreatable group of patients, with good short-term results. The long-term results were initially disappointing but are improving as techniques improve.

Balloon valvoplasty is also used in the treatment of Mitral and Pulmonary Stenoses, in both of which the initial results are very good and the long-term results so far are also good. Balloon dilatation is also of use in the dilatation of arterial stenoses (almost anywhere in the body), surgical shunts, coarctation or re-coarctation, some vascular surgical anastomoses, biliary and oesophageal strictures.

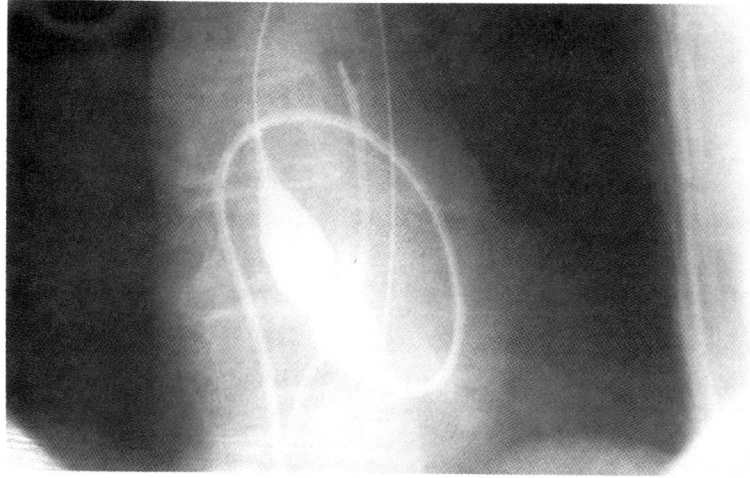

Figure 12*b*

CARDIOVASCULAR SYSTEM

Case 13

This 37-year-old patient has been followed up for a cardiac abnormality for many years. He gets short of breath on exertion and occasionally has been noticed to be slightly dusky, particularly on exertion.

This is his chest radiograph. What abnormalities are shown and what is the likely cause?

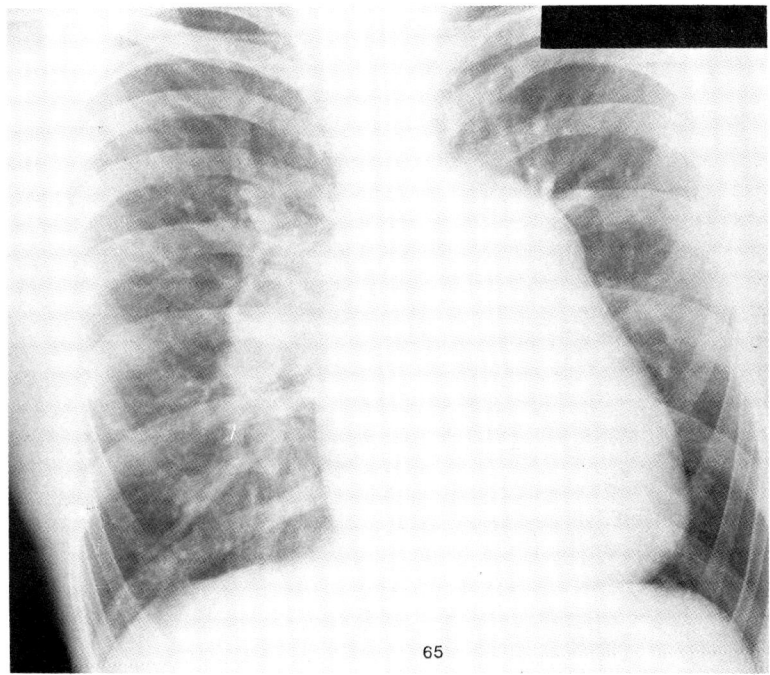

Figure 13

The cardiac abnormalities are marked enlargement of the main and proximal right and left pulmonary arteries, a heart with a transverse diameter at the upper limit of normal and small peripheral pulmonary arteries. The orientation of the ribs is abnormal with horizontal posterior and vertical anterior portions which suggests that the patient has pectus excavatum. Although pectus excavatum may cause the main pulmonary artery to be prominent the main pulmonary artery in this patient is far too large for this to be the explanation.

The large central pulmonary arteries and small peripheral pulmonary arteries suggest that this patient has Pulmonary Arterial Hypertension. In an adult male patient of this age the possible causes include Eisenmenger reaction, which could be due to a VSD, ASD or PDA, or rarely Thromboembolic Pulmonary Hypertension or Idiopathic Pulmonary Hypertension. The latter two diagnoses are more common in women. In this patient the very large main pulmonary artery would also make the last two diagnoses unlikely. In a patient with an Eisenmenger PDA the duct should be visible and is often calcified. In cases of ASD with a significant shunt the heart is usually enlarged until the Eisenmenger reaction sets in, and then the heart returns to a normal size. However, then the pulmonary artery enlargement usually extends further into the lobar pulmonary arteries than is the case here. The normal heart size and pulmonary artery enlargement confined to the more central pulmonary arteries seen here is typical but not diagnostic of an Eisenmenger VSD and this was the diagnosis proved by cardiac catheterization in this patient. Echocardiography would be a less invasive investigation but in adults it can be difficult to perform a complete examination, especially if the chest is deformed.

CARDIOVASCULAR SYSTEM

Case 14

This young child is cyanosed. What does this chest radiograph show? What are the differential diagnoses? What further investigations are required?

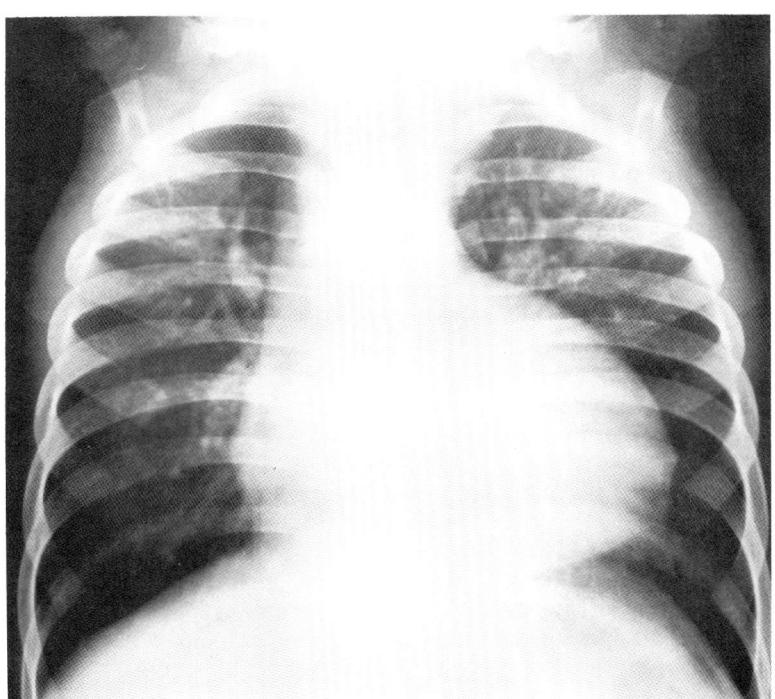

Figure 14

The heart is slightly enlarged (CTR 63 per cent) with an elevated cardiac apex and a right-sided aortic arch. There is a hollow pulmonary bay and the branching pattern of the pulmonary vessels is irregular and uneven. The cardiac configuration is suggestive of Pulmonary Atresia with a VSD, in which the heart tends to be larger than in Fallot's Tetralogy. This is in spite of the exclusion of this condition from some textbook lists of causes of pulmonary oligaemia and cardiomegaly (although the degree of cardiomegaly is usually only mild if present). The cardiac configuration (a good example of a 'coeur en sabot' in this case) and the presence of a right aortic arch would be consistent with both Fallot's Tetralogy and pulmonary atresia with a VSD (the cardiac configuration in isolated pulmonary atresia is different and the presence of a VSD should be specified when giving this differential diagnosis). A right-sided aortic arch is found in 25–30 per cent of cases of Fallot's Tetralogy and pulmonary atresia with VSD. It is also found in approximately 10 per cent of cases of tricuspid atresia which might be included in the differential diagnosis of cyanosis with oligaemia, but which is usually associated with a more rounded, less elevated, cardiac apex. The abnormal pulmonary vessels are consistent with the abnormal bronchopulmonary circulation which arises from the aorta in this type of pulmonary atresia.

Other causes of cyanotic heart disease with oligaemic lung fields and cardiomegaly include severe pulmonary stenosis (with an ASD), Ebstein's anomaly, Uhl's anomaly and single ventricle with pulmonary stenosis. None of these alternative diagnoses are associated with this cardiac configuration or a right-sided aortic arch.

Further investigation should include echocardiography, to confirm the diagnosis, and angiography to demonstrate the pulmonary blood supply, and to assess the possibility of surgical palliation.

CARDIOVASCULAR SYSTEM

Case 15

This is an apical four-chamber view from an echocardiogram on a child awaiting surgery for cyanotic congenital heart disease. What does it show? What are the usual abnormalities seen on chest radiographs in this condition?

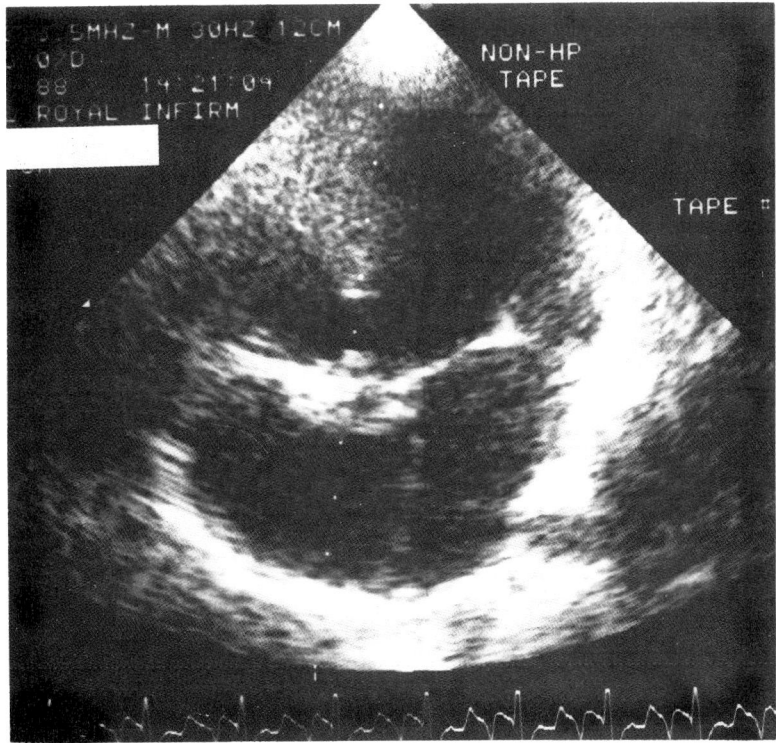

Figure 15a

The echocardiogram shows a normal thickness mitral valve but there is a thick shelf of tissue where the tricuspid valve should be. This represents the thickened mass of AV sulcus tissue seen in patients with Tricuspid Atresia. In addition there is a perimembranous VSD and no interatrial septum is visible. The interatrial septum is not always visible on this view and an ASD should not be diagnosed on the basis of an apical view only. In patients with tricuspid atresia there must be an ASD to allow outflow from the right atrium. The angiographic appearances are shown in *Fig. 15b* in which a left ventricular injection shows the aorta and, through a VSD, the pulmonary artery. There has been mitral regurgitation which has opacified both the atria and outlines the thick mass of AV sulcus tissue(↑), in which the right coronary artery can be seen, which has replaced the tricuspid valve.

The chest radiograph in tricuspid atresia usually shows a normal-size heart, until heart failure develops, and pulmonary oligaemia, unless there is a very large VSD. The pulmonary bay is usually small with small proximal pulmonary arteries. The cardiac apex may be rounded and elevated due to right atrial enlargement to the left, which displaces the right ventricle to the left. There is a right-sided aortic arch in up to 10 per cent cases.

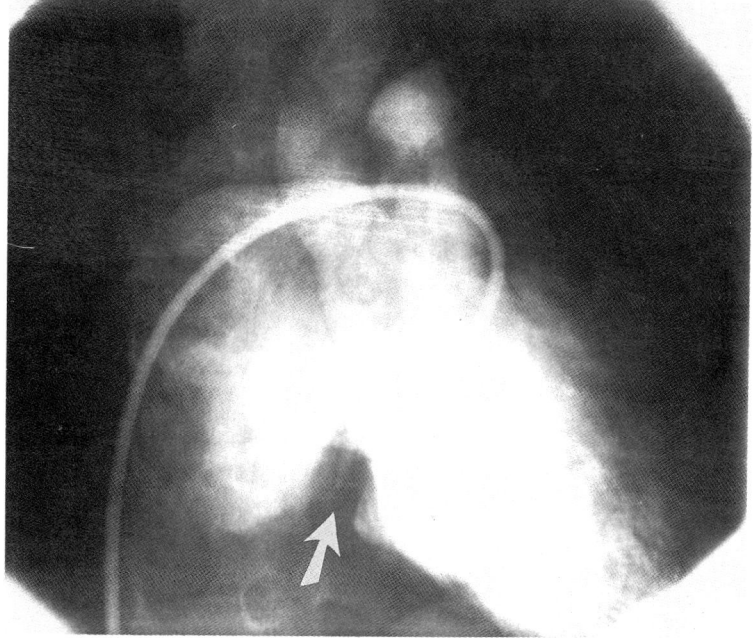

Figure 15*b*

Case 16

This investigation was performed on a 15-year-old girl who was well but had a murmur.

What is the investigation? What does it show and what conditions may be associated with this appearance?

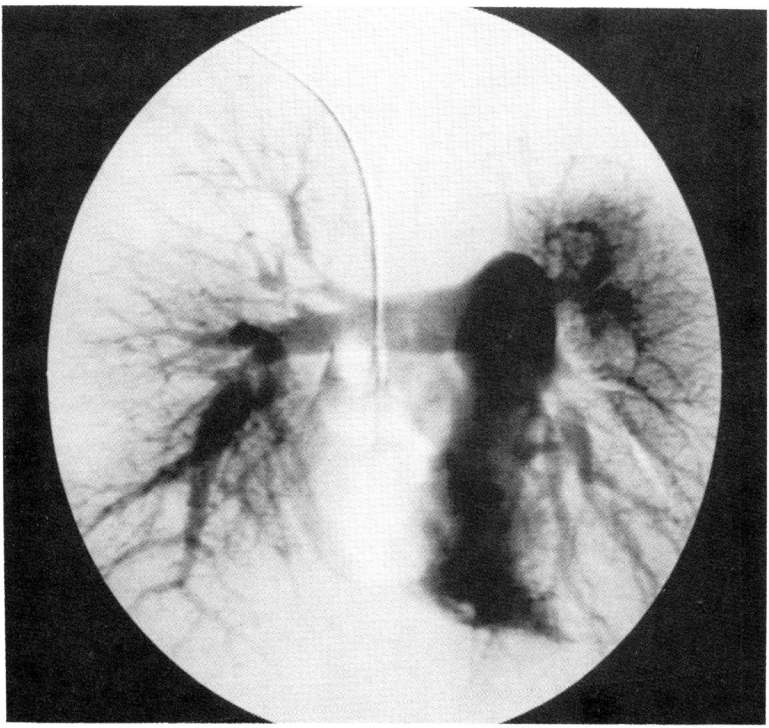

Figure 16

This is an Intravenous Digital Subtraction (i.v. DSA) Pulmonary Angiogram. Note the course of the central venous catheter used for the injection into the right atrium which indicates that this is an intravenous study rather than an intra-arterial study.

The angiogram shows Stenoses of the Peripheral Pulmonary Arteries, which are particularly well shown in the right upper lobe. This was an isolated finding in this case but pulmonary artery stenosis may be associated with the Maternal Rubella Syndrome, Ehlers–Danlos Syndrome or Infantile Hypercalcaemia, when there may also be supravalvar aortic stenosis. When these two conditions occur together they may be associated with abnormal facies and mental retardation. Proximal stenosis of the pulmonary arteries is also commonly found in Fallot's Tetralogy and can be associated with valvar pulmonary stenosis.

Pulmonary artery stenosis may be central, involving the origins of the right and left pulmonary arteries; peripheral involving the origins of the lobar or segmental vessels; or generalized, when it amounts to a general paucity of development of all of the pulmonary arteries.

Peripheral pulmonary stenoses are difficult to demonstrate by methods other than angiography, i.v. DSA can be performed quickly and safely on outpatients and gives very good definition of the abnormal areas.

CARDIOVASCULAR SYSTEM

Case 17

This is the chest radiograph of a young man who was admitted with sudden onset of chest pain, which was diagnosed as being due to a left pneumothorax. This chest radiograph (in the AP projection) was taken after insertion of a chest drain to relieve the pneumothorax. What are the abnormal radiographic features and what are the likely causes?

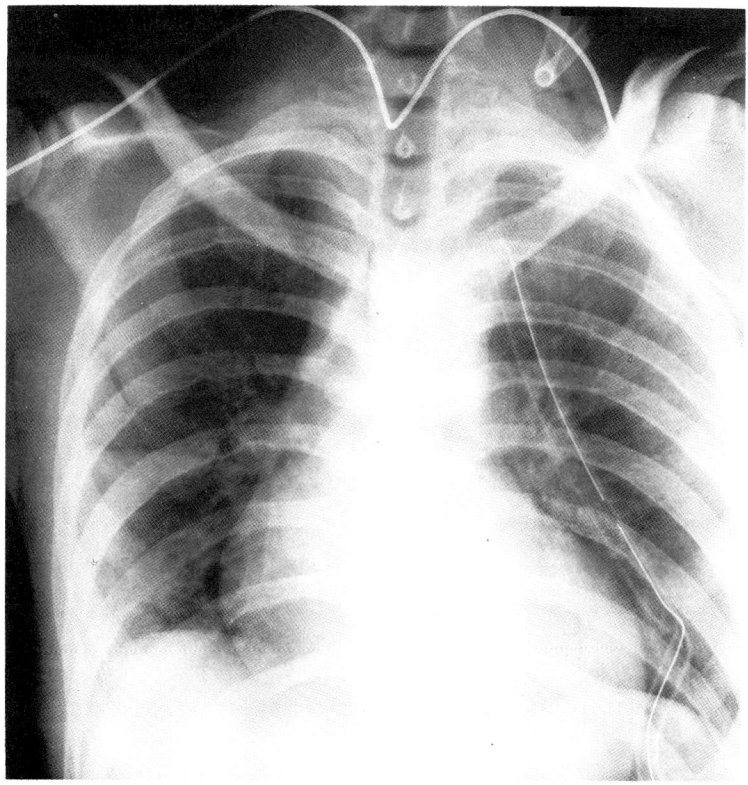

Figure 17

There is an intercostal chest drain in what appears to be a satisfactory position with no residual pneumothorax. There is surgical emphysema at the base of the neck on the left, which is not unusual following the insertion of a chest drain. Even making allowance for the AP projection the heart is large and there is bilateral inferior rib notching.

This was an unexpected finding and in this case was due to the most common cause of inferior rib notching, that is Coarctation of the Aorta. Although coarctation of the aorta has a number of other radiological signs (pre-stenotic dilatation, post-stenotic dilatation, left ventricular prominence) inferior rib notching is the most useful sign in adolescent and adult patients. The presence of rib notching in a patient with coarctation implies that there is a significant gradient across the coarctation. Unfortunately the rib notching persists after surgical correction and is therefore not a useful indicator of re-coarctation following surgery. The severity of coarctation can be determined clinically, by Doppler or angiography, although the latter is usually best accomplished using i.v. DSA unless pressure measurements are also required. The investigation of patients with coarctation is discussed in more detail in Case 10.

There are many causes of inferior rib notching of which coarctation of the aorta is by far the commonest. Other causes include aortic obstruction (by thrombosis, severe atheromatous disease, Takayasu's disease and other similar arteritic diseases), severe cyanotic congenital heart disease (including pulmonary atresia, and Fallot's Tetralogy), vena caval obstruction (superior or inferior), vascular malformations (particularly arteriovenous fistulae of the chest wall), neurofibromatosis and surgery (usually following a Blalock–Taussig shunt when the rib notching is seen on the side of the shunt). Other causes of inferior rib notching (hyperparathyroidism, extramedullary haemopoiesis) seldom cause confusion. Although the list of causes of rib notching is long, in practice the diagnosis is usually coarctation of the aorta when the notching is bilateral. If there is a right-sided aortic arch and unilateral rib notching the diagnosis is likely to be either Fallot's Tetralogy or Pulmonary Atresia palliated by a Blalock–Taussig shunt.

CARDIOVASCULAR SYSTEM

Case 18

This is the chest radiograph of a young child who was waiting for surgery. She is becoming increasingly cyanosed and is growing slowly. What does this radiograph show and what is the differential diagnosis? There are a number of features which suggest one particular diagnosis. What is it?

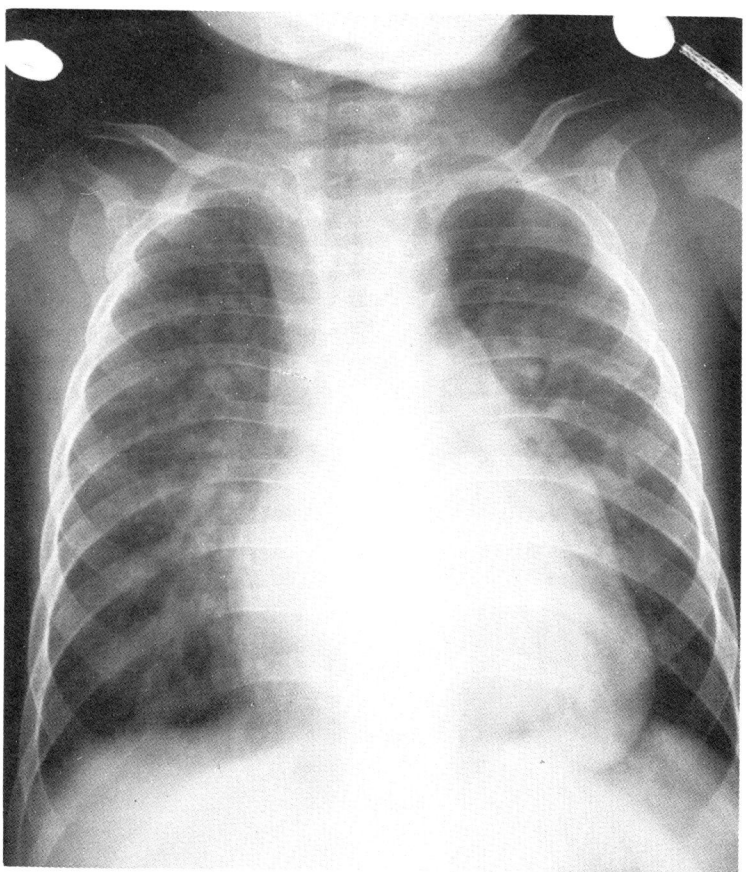

Figure 18

The heart is slightly enlarged and there is an unusual mediastinal outline. There is a long gentle bulge on the left mediastinal border at a site where the left atrial appendage is usually seen. However, this bulge is too long to be the left atrial appendage, enlargement of which is usually associated with mitral valve disease and therefore is rare in children. The main pulmonary artery can be seen above this but it is difficult to distinguish the ascending aorta, which is not visible in its usual position. There is also pulmonary plethora.

The important differential diagnoses of pulmonary plethora visible on a chest radiograph in a child with cyanotic heart disease include:
1. Transposition of the great arteries (usually with a narrow upper mediastinum).
2. Total anomalous pulmonary venous drainage (with a prominent ascending cardinal vein visible on chest radiography in the supracardiac type).
3. Truncus arteriosus (usually with a prominent ascending and arch of aorta); 50 per cent are associated with a right-sided aortic arch.
4. Tricuspid atresia with a VSD with no restriction of flow through the VSD and an obligatory ASD. An uncommon cause of plethora.
5. Single Ventricle. In single ventricle the aorta and main pulmonary artery are often abnormally related, either lying side by side or completely transposed. As in this case when the great arteries are transposed in association with single ventricle the aorta arises anterior and to the left of the pulmonary artery. On the chest radiograph it is seen as a long curving opacity arising above the left heart border and sweeping up to the aortic arch. Echocardiography confirms the diagnosis.

Case 19

This patient was admitted to hospital as an emergency and subsequently had this investigation. At the time of this investigation his chest radiograph was reported to be normal. What is this investigation? Describe the nature of *Figure* 19 *a* and 19 *b*. What do these images show and what is the most likely diagnosis? What is the differential diagnosis of this appearance and which diagnoses are relevant in this patient?

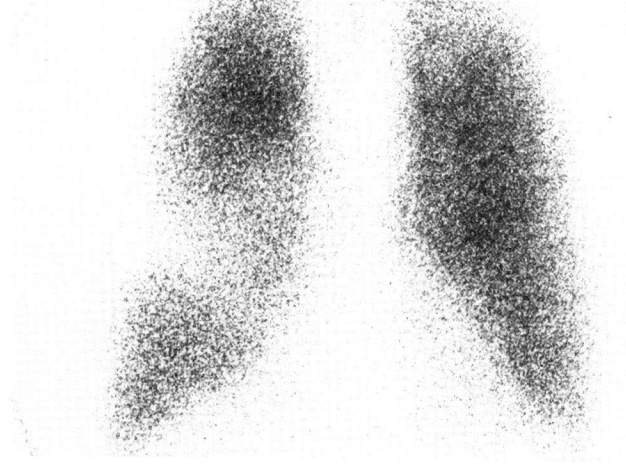

Figure 19 *a*

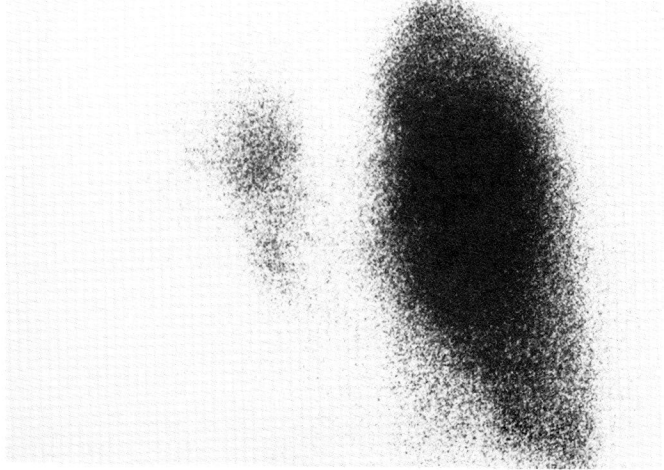

Figure 19 *b*

This is a Ventilation Perfusion Lung Scan with the anterior ventilation image shown in *Fig.* 19*a* (note the activity from the inhaled krypton in the trachea) and the anterior perfusion image shown in *Fig.* 19*b*. The images show a small right mid-zone ventilation defect but a very extensive perfusion defect involving almost all of the right lung, except for a small segment of the right upper lobe. In a patient who is acutely ill and who has been reported to have a normal chest radiograph the likely diagnosis is a Large Pulmonary Embolus. Opinions on the usefulness and sensitivity of the chest radiograph in the diagnosis of pulmonary embolism vary. Often under these circumstances the chest radiograph at the time of presentation is normal but abnormalities often develop after a short time. These are often clearer in retrospect, especially when the results of the lung scan are known. The chest radiograph is essential for interpreting the lung scan.

The differential diagnosis of this appearance is small. Although many conditions can cause perfusion defects (including chronic airways disease, tumours, pneumonia, tuberculosis, lung abscess, fibrosis and hypoplasia of the lung) the majority also produce matching ventilation defects and diagnostic changes on the chest radiograph. Occasionally it is possible for a tumour or other local disease process (such as fibrosis and radiation pneumonitis) to involve preferentially a pulmonary artery and cause an unmatched perfusion defect, and therefore mimic the appearance of pulmonary embolism. In the clinical situation described in this case the diagnosis should not be in doubt and further investigation by angiography is only indicated if thrombolytic therapy or thrombectomy are being considered.

Case 20

What does this M-mode echocardiogram show? What other echocardiographic abnormalities can this condition produce? How would you assess its severity?

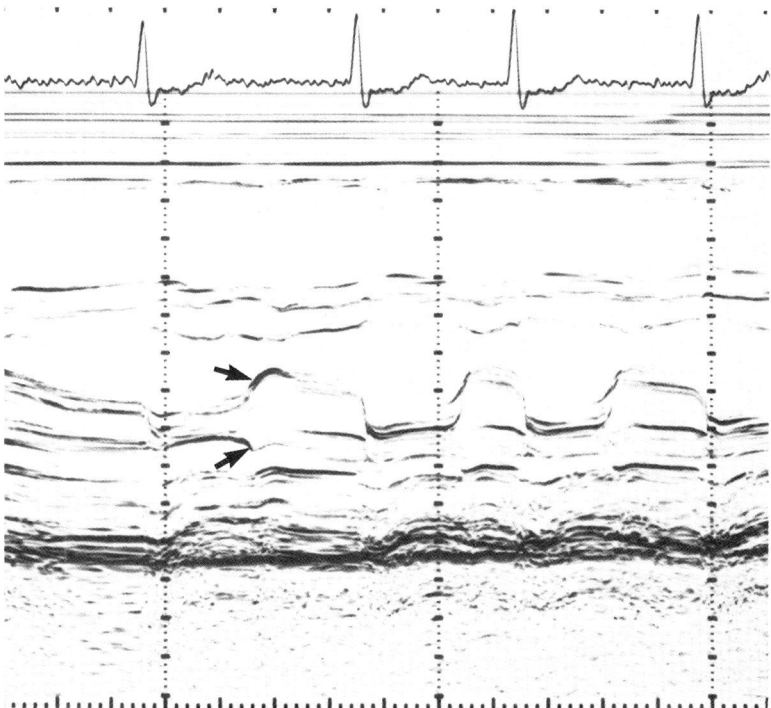

Figure 20

The echocardiogram shows thickening of the mitral valve cusps (→), particularly the anterior cusp, with slow closure of the valve during diastole (reduced diastolic closure rate—DCR) and anterior motion of the posterior cusp during diastole. These are the features of Mitral Stenosis. Other echocardiographic features include Calcification of the Mitral Valve, Slow Diastolic Filling of the Left Ventricle (best appreciated by M-mode echocardiography), Large Left Atrium and occasionally Left Atrial Thrombus. On 2-D echocardiography the mitral valve orifice seen in the short axis view is small, although this is not a reliable method for measuring the severity of the stenosis. There may also be evidence of pulmonary hypertension as indicated by Abnormal Pulmonary Valve Motion, Dilated Right Ventricle and Doppler evidence of Pulmonary and Tricuspid Regurgitation.

The severity of mitral stenosis is best measured non-invasively by Doppler measurement of the pressure half-time (*see Fig. 4b*). In this calculation the time for the pressure gradient across the valve to fall by 50 percent (pressure half-time expressed in milliseconds) is measured and can be related to the valve area (mitral valve area = 220/pressure half-time). Although there are instances when this method is not wholly reliable or where other conditions may mimic the flow pattern of mitral stenosis (particularly aortic regurgitation), in most patients this provides a valuable method for assessing the severity of mitral stenosis. Using Doppler it is also possible to estimate the peak and mean gradients across the valve, although these values are of less use in assessing the severity of stenosis unless the cardiac output is also known. In some equivocal cases cardiac catheterization with measurement of left and right heart pressures, with cardiac output, may allow more confident assessment of the stenosis and also allow assessment of any coronary artery disease prior to surgery.

Case 21

This is a contrast-enhanced CT scan from a patient who had an aortic valve replacement for aortic stenosis five years previously, which was complicated by a superficial wound infection. What does this image show? What is its probable significance in this patient? What other conditions may be associated with this appearance? What are the useful alternative methods for showing this abnormality?

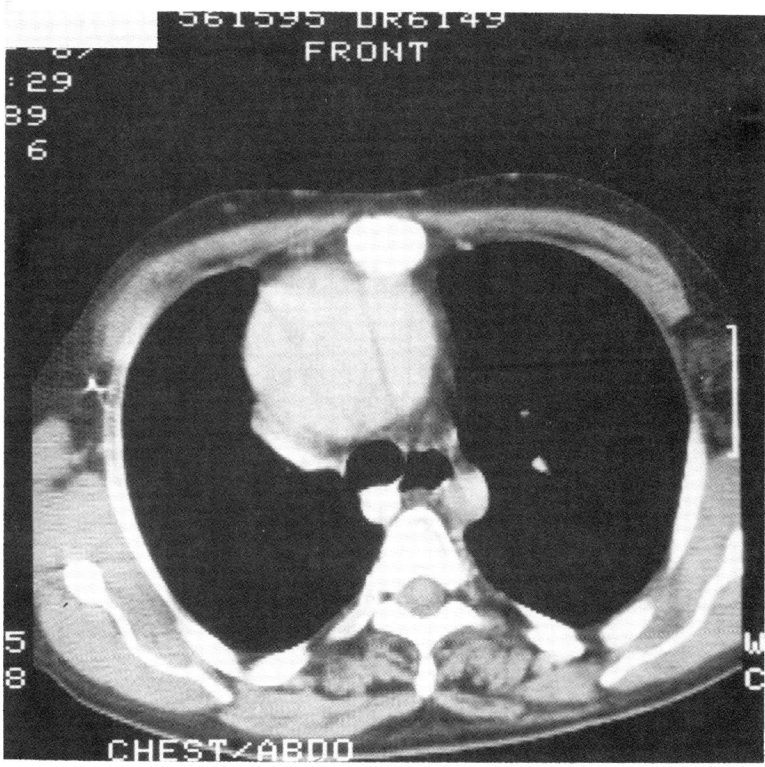

Figure 21*a*

This scan image shows that the ascending aorta is dilated and there is a dissection flap within it. The descending aorta is not dilated and there is no dissection flap visible within it. In this particular patient the development of the ascending aortic dissection is most probably related either to damage of the aorta at the time of his previous surgery or the subsequent wound infection, which is a well recognized association with aortic dissections following bypass grafting and valve replacement.

Many other conditions are related to aortic dissection, the most important of these include: Hypertension, Atherosclerosis, Pregnancy, Marfan's Syndrome, Chest Trauma, Coarctation, Bicuspid Aortic Valve and various rarer connective tissue disorders such as Ehlers–Danlos Syndrome.

The useful alternatives for demonstrating this type of lesion are echocardiography (which is limited to examining the ascending aorta, part of the arch and abdominal aorta), MRI (*Fig.* 21*b* shows the MRI scan taken at the same level as the CT scan in this patient) and angiography. In this particular case angiography was unhelpful due to dilution of the contrast medium in the huge false lumen. MRI was the most useful investigation in this patient as it clearly showed the relationship of the dissection to the origins of the head and neck vessels, an area which was not clearly shown by the CT.

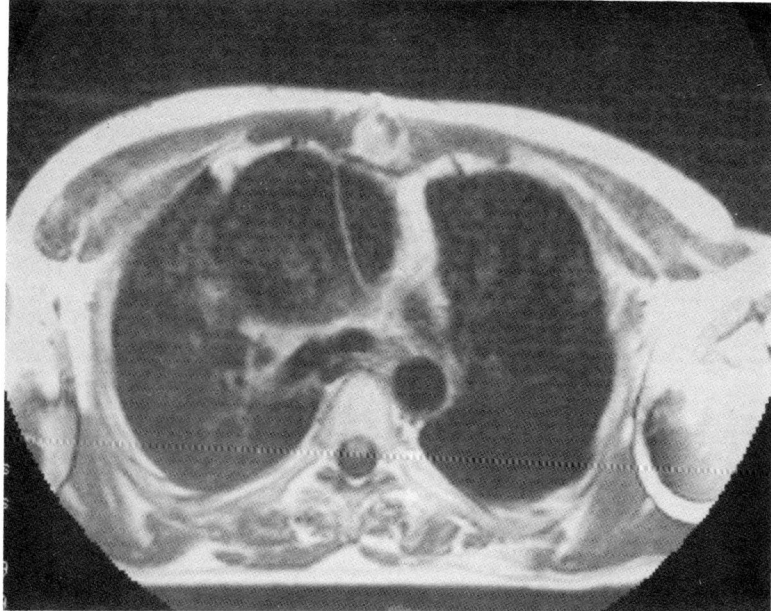

Figure 21*b*

Case 22

This image was acquired a few seconds after a femoral artery injection of contrast medium. What has been done to this image? What does it show? What are the possible differential diagnoses?

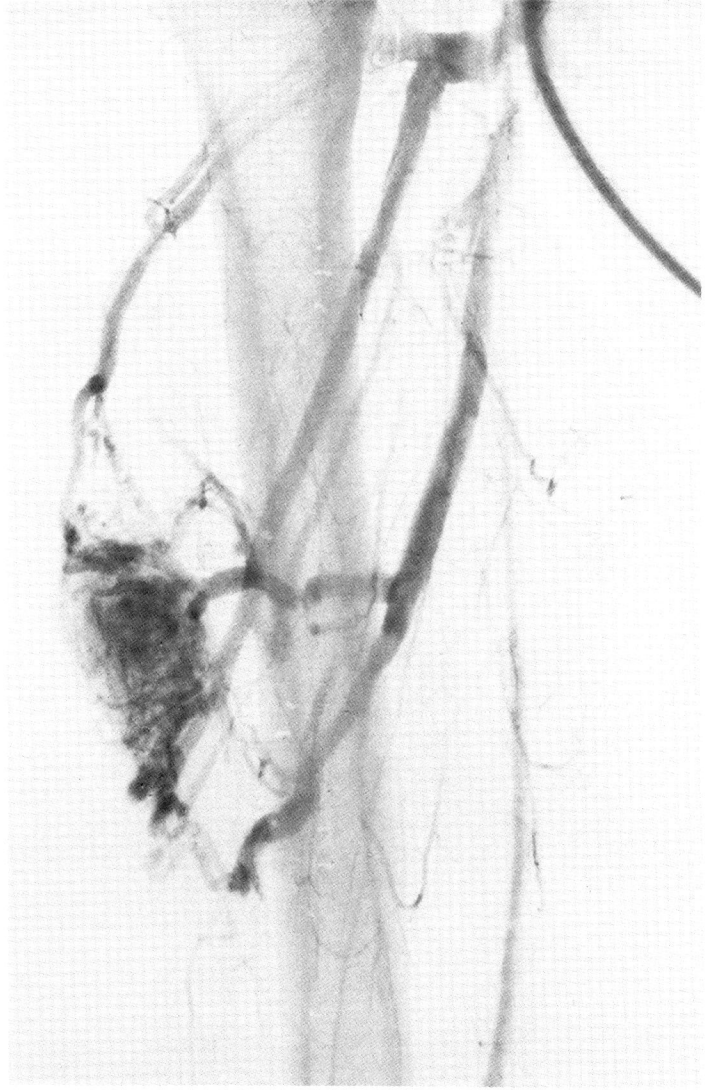

Figure 22*a* (By courtesy of Professor D. J. Allison)

This image has been produced by performing Photographic Subtraction on the original angiographic image. This uses the conventional angiographic film and a control film to produce the subtracted image. This is unlike DSA which uses computerized subtraction of digital images to produce a similar type of image, although the resolution of the DSA image is not as good. The image shows a very vascular localized lesion in the thigh with abnormal vessels running into it. Judging by the lack of contrast in the proximal femoral artery in this picture it seems likely that the abnormal vessels are veins (this was confirmed by examining the rest of the arteriogram). Large feeding arteries were seen on an earlier exposure.

There is a relatively small differential diagnosis for this appearance of a localized, very vascular soft tissue tumour. Possibilities include:

1. Vascular metastases (the likeliest sources being thyroid carcinoma and hypernephroma).
2. Arteriovenous malformation (as shown in *Fig.* 22*b* which is a DSA image of an arteriovenous malformation in the upper arm).
3. Angiosarcoma (the diagnosis in the case shown in *Fig.* 22*a*).
4. Haemangiopericytoma.

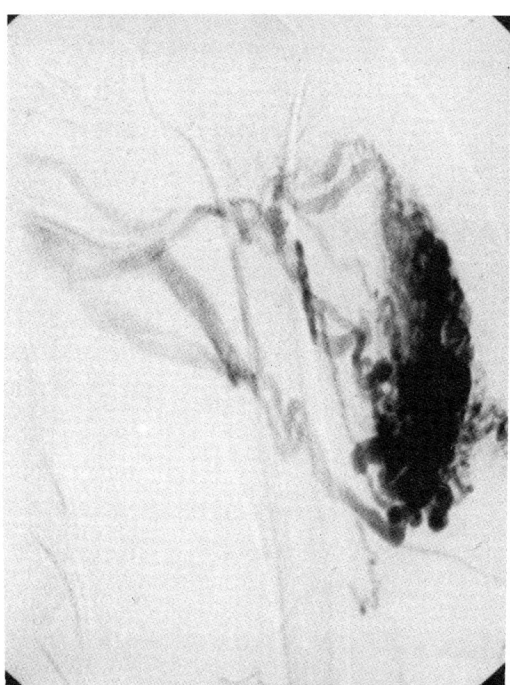

Figure 22*b* (By courtesy of Professor D. J. Allison)

Case 23

This is the chest radiograph of a 60-year-old male patient who was being investigated for hypertension. What are the radiographic features of importance on this film and what is the likely diagnosis? What are the alternative diagnoses and what other features might support these less likely differentials? What is the significance of the most likely diagnosis? What further investigations may be required?

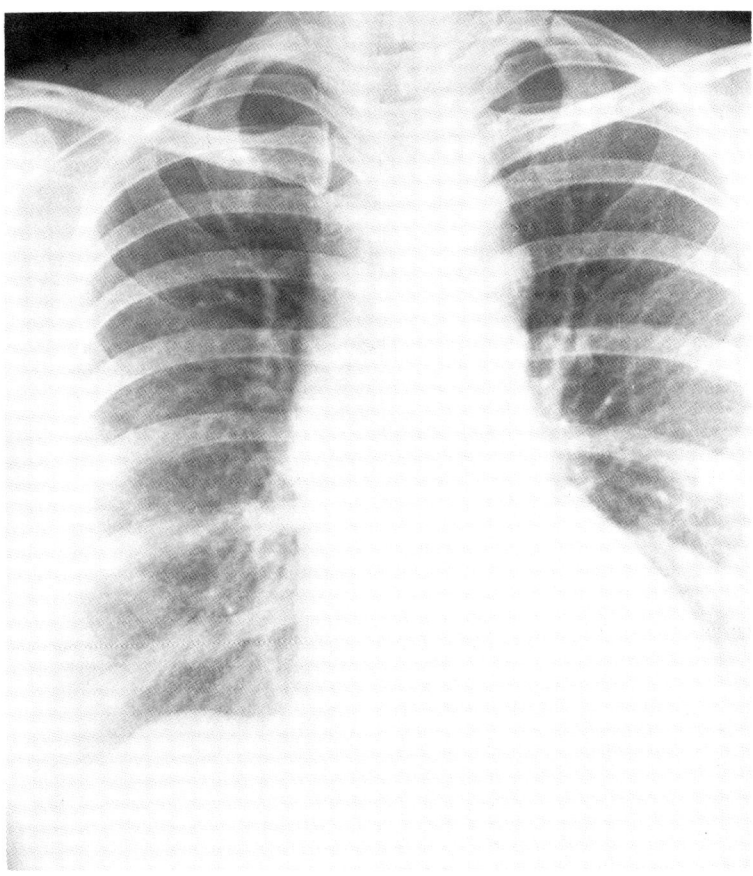

Figure 23

There is an abnormal prominence and unusual configuration of the aortic arch. The aortic arch is high, wide and there is a second prominence of the descending aorta below the arch. The heart is enlarged but the lung fields are normal. The ribs are normal and in particular there is no rib notching. This appearance of two aortic knuckles, one high and one low, in the absence of rib notching suggests the diagnosis of Pseudocoarctation. The large heart is consistent with the stated diagnosis of hypertension.

The differential diagnoses include True Coarctation and Mediastinal Tumours, such as secondary deposits in lymph nodes and thymoma. In patients with true coarctation there should be rib notching to indicate that there is a significant gradient across the coarctation. If there has been surgical repair there is often at least one abnormal rib to indicate the site of a lateral thoracotomy. In patients with a mediastinal mass there may be evidence of tracheal compression, lymphadenopathy elsewhere on the chest radiograph or bone involvement.

If there is doubt about the diagnosis further investigations should be aimed at excluding coarctation and mediastinal masses. Coarctation can usually be excluded clinically but if there is significant doubt angiography (preferably by i.v. DSA) or MRI will show the aortic arch anatomy. In pseudocoarctation angiography shows elongation and kinking of the aorta without significant narrowing and without chest wall collaterals. In patients where a mediastinal mass is considered as a differential CT is a satisfactory method for examining the mediastinum. MRI, where it is available, can be used to exclude both coarctation and mediastinal tumours.

Case 24

This mentally subnormal patient was admitted for investigation of slowly increasing shortness of breath and signs of right heart failure. Frontal chest radiographs showed no abnormality within the lungs. This was the lateral chest radiograph. What does this show and what is the likely cause of her symptoms and signs? What further investigations might you consider to establish the diagnosis and what problems might be encountered in using them?

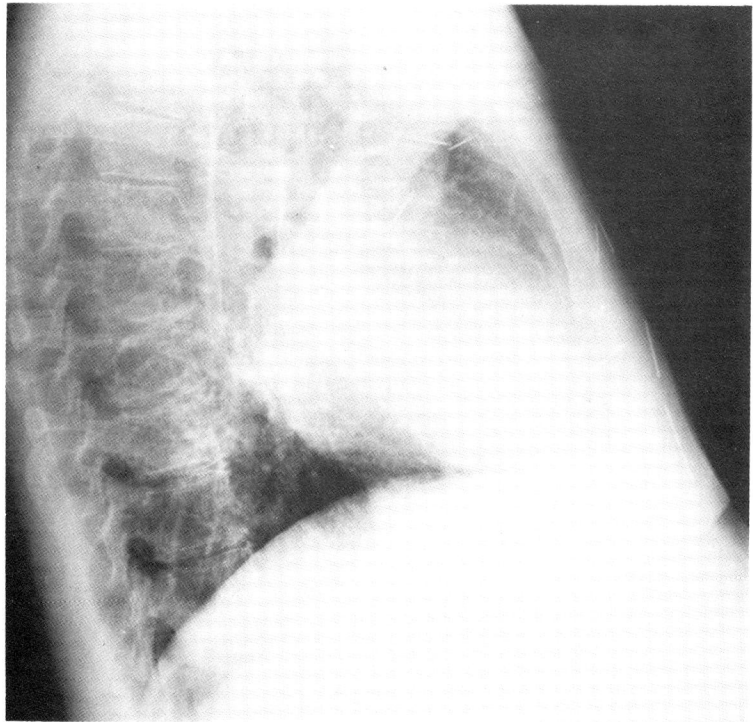

Figure 24

There are several straight thin metallic density objects projected over the anterior chest wall and the anterior and middle mediastinum. These are the shape and size of needles. This is indeed what they were. The patient has symptoms and signs of pericardial constriction and you are told that there is no abnormality in the lungs, which rules out a pneumothorax or pulmonary infection as a cause of her shortness of breath. With the symptoms and the presence of multiple sharp foreign bodies in the vicinity of the pericardium, Constrictive Pericarditis is a likely diagnosis, either resulting from repeated episodes of haemopericardium or pericardial infection, or both. Proving the diagnosis in a mentally retarded patient with self-mutilating tendencies could be difficult.

Echocardiography is probably the initial investigation of choice to determine if there is a pericardial effusion which requires drainage and to show signs of constriction (such as a small right ventricle or right ventricular diastolic collapse). It may be possible to estimate the pericardial thickness but other methods are usually required to do this. CT may be useful if the patient can be kept still during each scan. Artefacts from the needles may obscure some detail. MRI is a very good method for demonstrating pericardial disease but is contraindicated in this case. Sewing needles are usually magnetic and the pull on these from the magnet could cause them to migrate within the patient. Considering the close proximity of some of these to the heart, and in particular the coronary arteries running on the surface of the heart, the hazards presented by such migration could be considerable. Also examining mentally retarded patients in the confines of the MRI scanner, where good cooperation and a relaxed, stationary patient are essential, is often unrewarding unless a general anaesthetic is justified.

CARDIOVASCULAR SYSTEM 49

Case 25

This patient had surgery for a cardiac condition one year ago. What was (were) the likely underlying condition(s) which led to his surgery?
What other abnormalities are shown on this chest radiograph and what might have caused them?

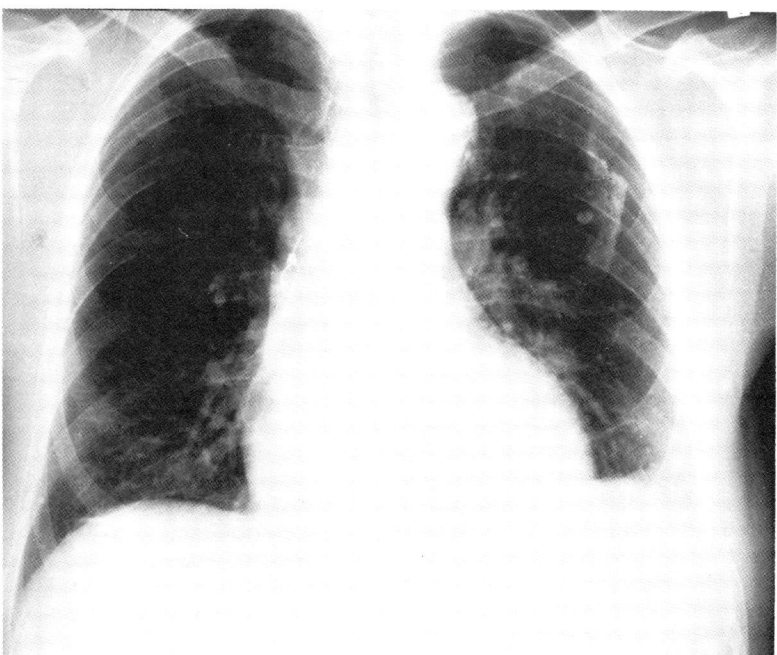

Figure 25a

This radiograph shows a slightly enlarged heart, a sternal suture, dilatation of the ascending aorta (shown by the position of the metal wire vein graft marker), slight elevation of the left hemidiaphragm, blunting of the left costophrenic angle (most probably due to pleural thickening in this case) and a large calcified pleural plaque projected over the left mid-zone. The presence of the vein graft marker indicates that the patient has had at least one Coronary Bypass Graft (to the right coronary artery from the position of the marker) but this cannot explain the prominence of the ascending aorta which is due to Post-Stenotic Dilatation above a Stenotic Aortic Valve, which was replaced by a Björk–Shiley valve (as shown on the lateral film, *Fig.* 25 *b*). Further pleural calcification is shown over the dome of the left hemidiaphragm and posterior chest wall. The surgery is too recent to be related to these pleural changes, which are characteristic of previous Empyema or Haemothorax. In this case the patient had had a Tuberculous Empyema.

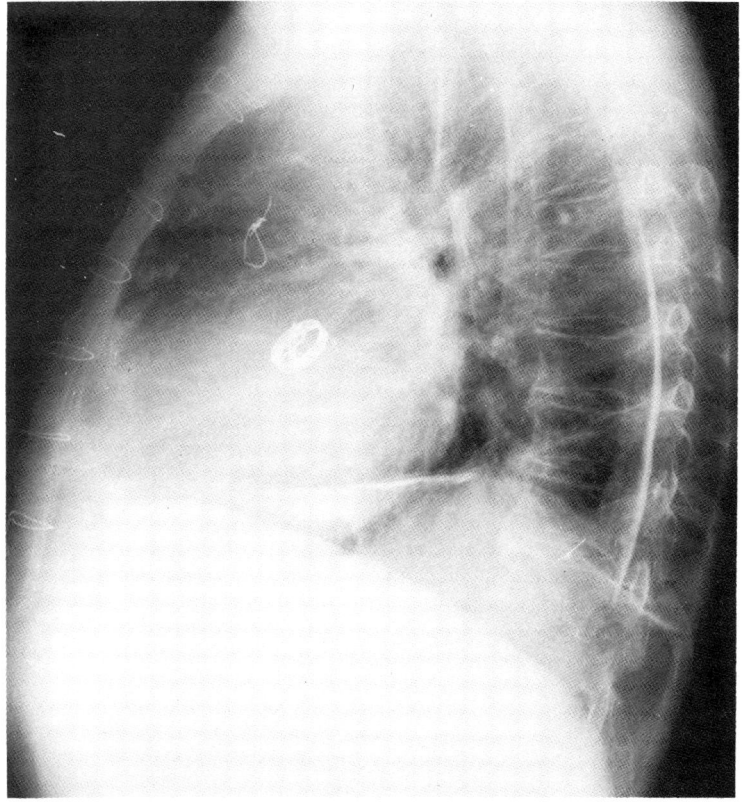

Figure 25 *b*

CARDIOVASCULAR SYSTEM

Case 26

What does the chest radiograph of this 56-year-old female patient show? What is the differential diagnosis and what is the most likely of these diagnoses? What confirmatory test would you perform to confirm the diagnosis?

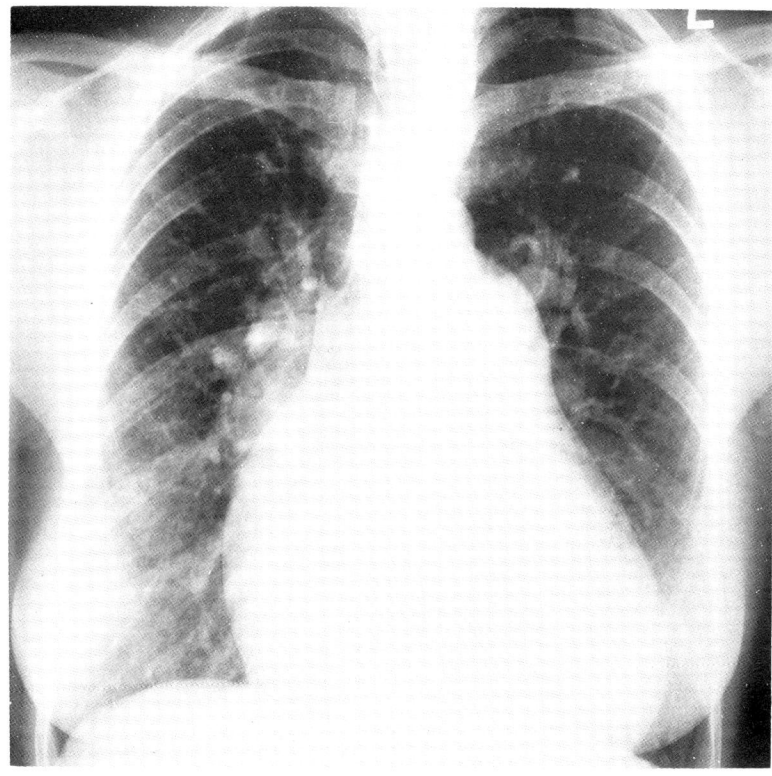

Figure 26

The abnormal features shown on this radiograph include a large heart, and large proximal arteries with the enlargement extending into some of the lobar pulmonary arteries. There is a relatively small aortic knuckle. The peripheral pulmonary arteries are small relative to the size of the proximal pulmonary arteries. These features suggest that there is a shunt with the development of a degree of pulmonary arterial hypertension (see discussion of Case 13). The possible differential diagnoses include ASD, VSD, PDA. At this age the last two are uncommon. In a VSD the heart may be enlarged but not often as large as this and the pulmonary artery enlargement does not often extend into the lobar pulmonary arteries, as it does in this case. The same applies to PDA which is often also visible and may cause enlargement of the aortic arch. The features shown on this picture are typical of an ASD (secundum type at this age) with pulmonary hypertension. However, it is unlikely that an Eisenmenger syndrome has developed yet as an Eisenmenger ASD is usually associated with a reduction in heart size towards normal. Adult patients with an ASD often have few symptoms and can present for the first time late in life with this sort of chest radiograph.

An Echocardiogram is the next useful investigation to confirm the diagnosis and to give an estimate of pulmonary artery pressure (see discussion of Case 13).

CARDIOVASCULAR SYSTEM
Case 27

What is this investigation and what does it show? What are the contraindications to the use of this technique? What suitable alternative imaging methods are available to obtain this information and what is their accuracy?

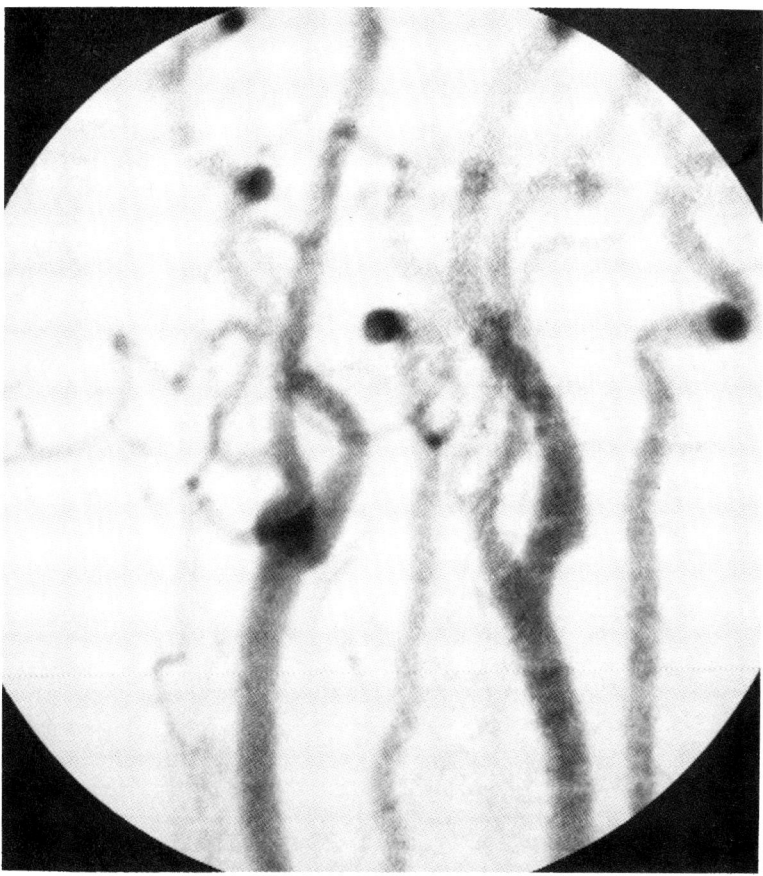

Figure 27a

This is an i.v. DSA Carotid Arteriogram taken in the left anterior oblique projection. There is a mild stenosis of the proximal left internal carotid artery equal to a reduction in luminal diameter of approximately 15 per cent. Measurements of this minor degree at this level can be difficult as there is normally some widening of the lumen of the artery at the level of the carotid bulb above the bifurcation, measured against the vessel above the bulb the stenosis is about 15 per cent.

The contraindications to i.v. DSA are related to those conditions which predispose to poor image quality and those conditions in which the administration of large doses of contrast media is contraindicated. The first group includes patients with Poor Cardiac Output, Occluded Vessels Proximal to the Area of Interest, Patients who are Unable to Cooperate and those with No Accessible Veins. The patients in whom the administration of contrast media is a relative or absolute contraindication include those with a History of Allergic Reactions, Asthma or other significant Atopic Conditions, Renal Impairment, Diabetes, Heart Failure and Advanced Age.

Extracranial carotid artery disease can also be demonstrated at a greater risk to the patient by Intra-arterial Angiography but the best non-invasive alternative is Duplex Doppler, which in expert hands has an overall accuracy in excess of 90 per cent compared to angiography. This is illustrated by *Fig.* 27 *b* which is a Duplex Doppler Scan from the same patient showing some spectral broadening (↑) in the deceleration phase of systole, indicating a stenosis of up to 15 per cent. Other Doppler methods and real time ultrasound are available but are generally less accurate in assessing the severity of a stenosis.

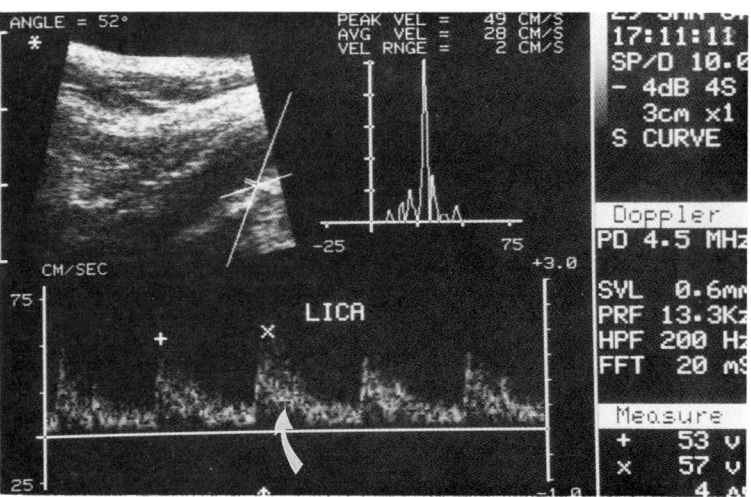

Figure 27 *b*

Case 28

This patient recently underwent an abdominal operation. What does this chest radiograph show? What is the likeliest diagnosis and what are the alternatives? What are the possible chest radiograph findings in this condition? What further investigations are available to confirm the diagnosis and what are their drawbacks?

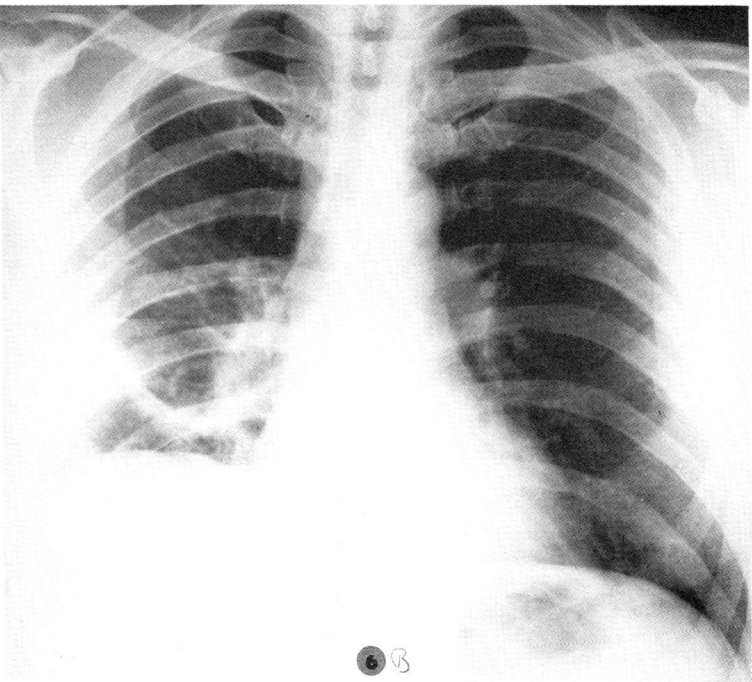

Figure 28

The chest radiograph shows elevation of the right hemidiaphragm and a triangular opacity in the right lower zone with its base adjacent to the chest wall. There is no significant mediastinal shift and the left lung appears normal. This is a characteristic if uncommon appearance of a Pulmonary Infarct due to Acute Pulmonary Embolism. Possible but less likely alternatives include postoperative or infective collapse and consolidation. The radiographic changes found in acute pulmonary embolism include: Focal Oligaemia, Focal Consolidation (characteristically but uncommonly triangular shaped and pleural based as in this case), Pleural Effusion, Linear Collapse, Elevation of a Hemidiaphragm, Cardiomegaly and Pulmonary Artery Dilatation. A normal chest radiograph is often seen initially in acute pulmonary embolism but only a minority of patients will have a normal radiograph throughout.

The safest accurate way of making the diagnosis is with a ventilation perfusion lung scan (see discussion in Case 19). This requires the use of isotopes and a Gamma camera, which are not always available, especially out of normal working hours. Interpretation of the scans is often difficult, especially in the presence of chronic cardiorespiratory disease, and can require considerable skill. Pulmonary angiography is the other widely available technique for diagnosing pulmonary emboli. This is a method which may be more readily available than isotope scanning, particularly out of hours. It may be hazardous, particularly in patients with large emboli or pulmonary hypertension, and requires both radiological and radiographic skills which may not be available at all times. Interpretation, particularly in the presence of chronic cardiopulmonary disease and focal infarction, can be difficult. The use of angiography may be combined with thrombolytic therapy, which can be infused through the same catheter, and sequential angiograms to evaluate progress may be useful. In the rare situations where surgery is contemplated angiography is essential.

Case 29

This is the echocardiogram of a patient who complained of being unwell but was unable to give any more history in English. What does this show and what are the possible differential diagnoses which can cause this condition?

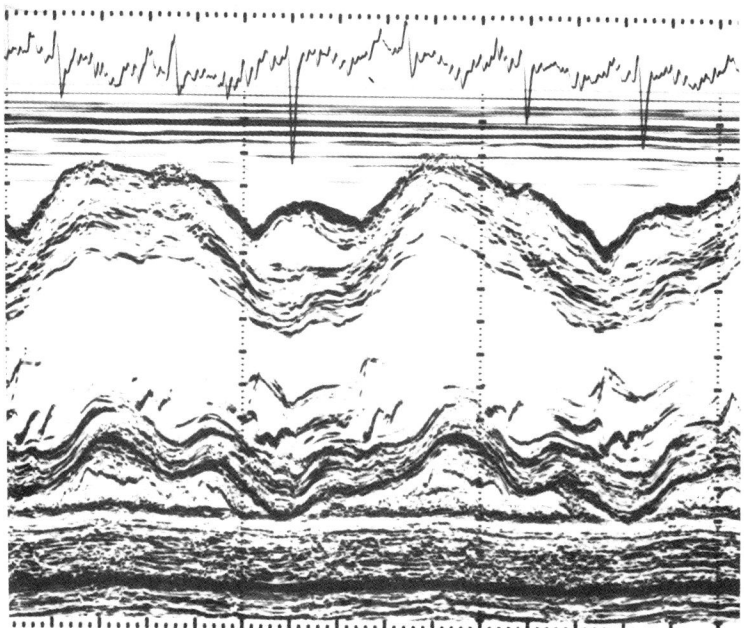

Figure 29a

This is an M-mode echogardiogram of the Left Ventricle at the level of the tips of the Mitral Valve Cusps. It shows the heart swinging around in a large echo-free space which is visible anteriorly and posteriorly. This is a Large Pericardial Effusion, which is particularly well seen anteriorly. This was confirmed by 2-D echocardiography (*Fig.* 29b, a subcostal view in the same patient) which also shows that the right ventricle (RV) is small and has a concave anterior wall (↓), which is an indication of compression in cardiac tamponade. This is a very large effusion (EFF) which should be easy to drain but in difficult cases 2-D echocardiography is also useful for guiding the tip of the aspirating needle into the effusion.

The important commoner causes of pericardial effusion include: Congestive Heart Failure, Dressler's Syndrome, Infective Pericarditis (including tuberculous, pyogenic, viral), Renal Failure, Rheumatoid Arthritis, Systemic Lupus Erythematosus and other similar multisystem diseases, Pericardial Malignancy (particularly spread from mediastinal malignancy), Cardiac Surgery/Chest Injury, Aortic Dissection, Cardiac Rupture (i.e. following myocardial infarction).

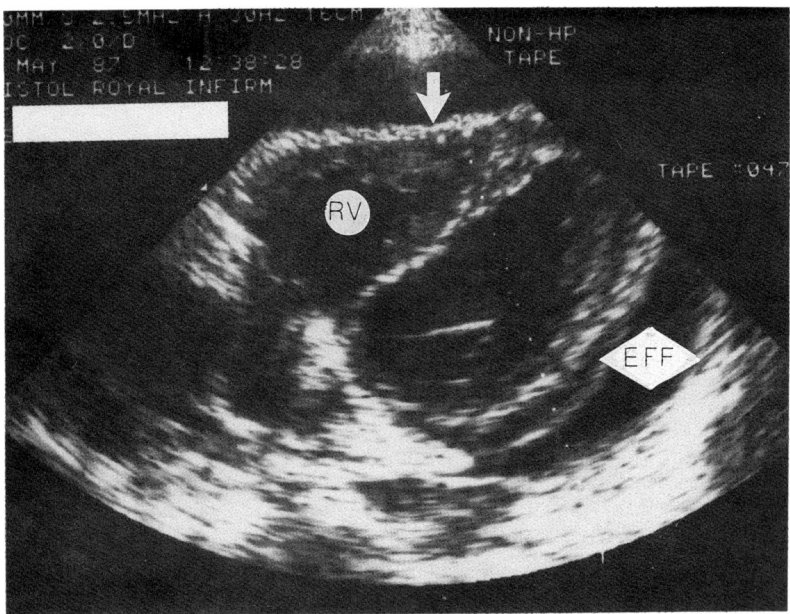

Figure 29b

Case 30

What is this venographic investigation and what does it show? What are the therapeutic implications of these findings? What alternative imaging methods are available to obtain this information?

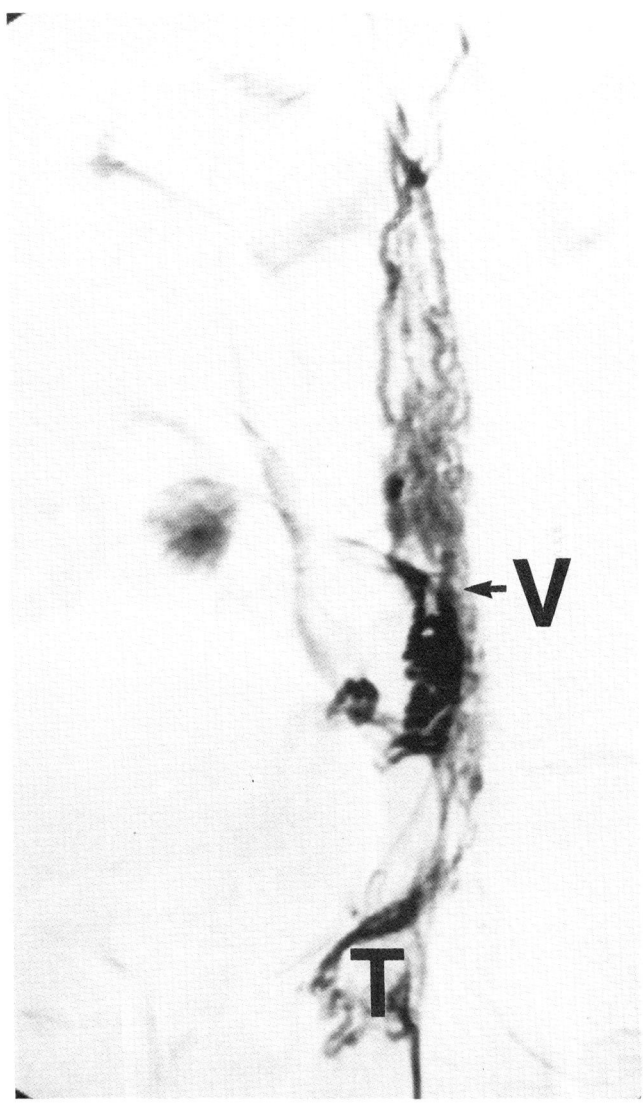

Figure 30*a* (By Courtesy of Professor A. P. Hemingway)

This is a DSA Left Testicular Venogram which shows an Incompletely Descended Left Testis (T) in the left inguinal canal and a very large Intra-abdominal Varicocele (V). The maldescended testis is at risk of injury in this site, may atrophy and is also at risk from torsion. The most important potential hazard is the increased risk of malignant changes in the maldescended testis, which requires orchidopexy in suitable cases, orchidectomy when this is not possible. The presence of a varicocele in this patient was probably of relatively little importance as the other testis was normal. Varicoceles may be a cause of infertility and are often best treated by embolization which, unlike surgery, has been shown to significantly improve fertility.

Alternative methods for demonstrating a maldescended testis include ultrasound (especially for a testis in the inguinal canal), CT and MRI (*Fig.* 30*b* shows a small testis in the scrotum which was not apparent on clinical examination). The ability of MRI to acquire coronal images is potentially very valuable in this context.

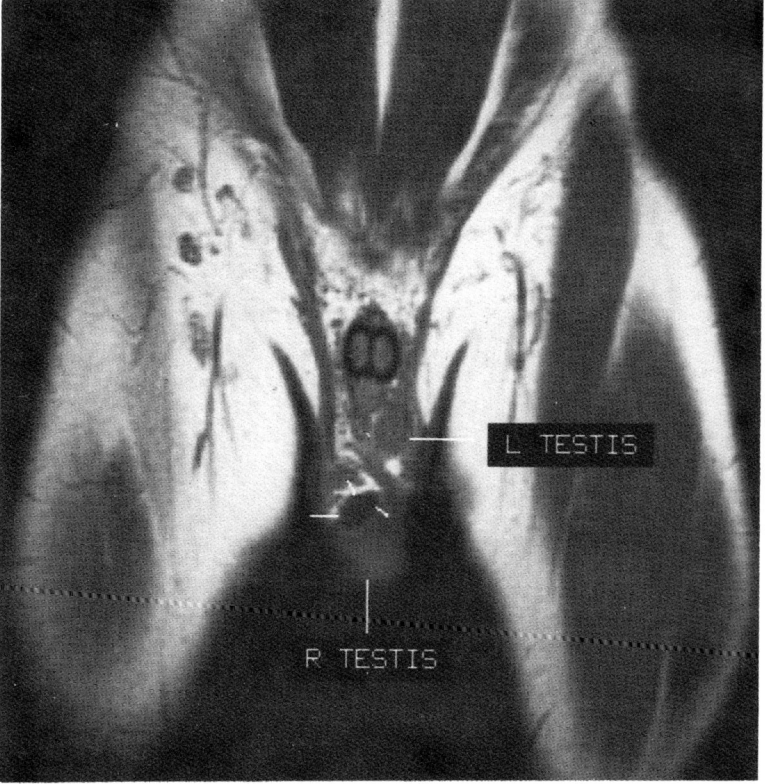

Figure 30*b*

Case 31

This is a selective left brachial arteriogram in a young man. What does it show and what are the possible causes? What are the complications? What possible treatment options are there?

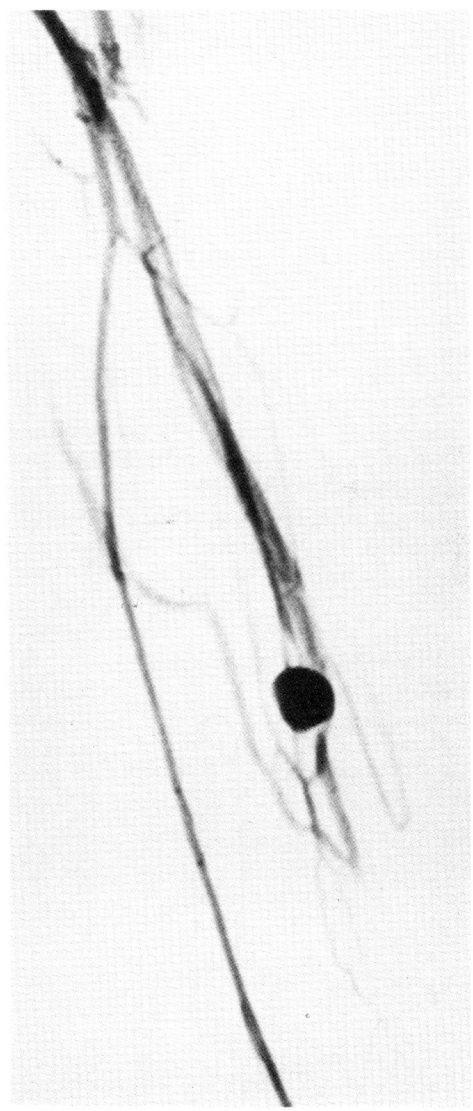

Figure 31 *a*

This DSA arteriogram shows simultaneous opacification of the radial and ulnar artery, several veins (including the basilic vein) and a large collection of contrast medium adjacent to the mid-radial artery. There is poor distal filling of the radial artery beyond the collection of contrast. The collection of contrast is a Radial Artery Aneurysm and the early venous filling indicates that there is also an Arteriovenous Fistula. The poor distal arterial filling indicates that there may be distal ischaemia.

Causes of an arteriovenous fistula of this type with aneurysm formation include:

1. Trauma (particularly fractures or penetrating injury, a knife wound in this case). Therapeutic or investigative procedures such as cardiac catheterization, angioplasty, biopsies and procedures on adjacent structures such as hip replacement and repair of fractures. Artificial shunts for haemodialysis may also be dilated (as well as stenosed, as in *Fig.* 31*b* which shows a dialysis shunt with two stenoses on the venous side and poor distal arterial flow). Rarely, congenital lesions can have this appearance.

2. Aneurysms in the absence of fistulae can also complicate cervical ribs, osteochondromas, use of crutches, pancreatitis, Ehlers–Danlos syndrome and other primary diseases of the arterial wall.

Aneurysms can rupture or thrombose, causing distal ischaemia, and act as a site of origin for distal emboli. Local pressure on nerves can cause weakness and paraesthesia.

Normally treatment is by resection with repair using a vein graft. In some difficult situations embolization may be a preferable alternative.

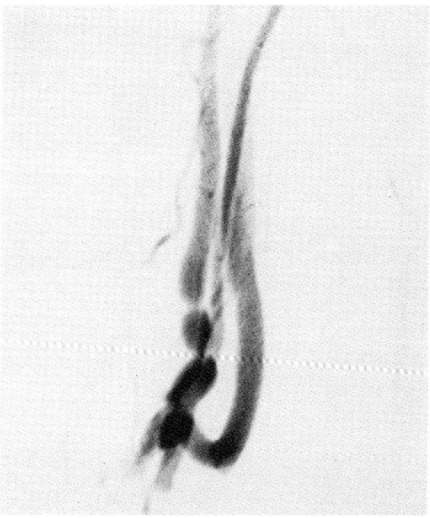

Figure 31*b*

Case 32

What abnormalities does this chest radiograph show? This radiographic appearance is strongly suggestive of one of two diagnoses. What are they?

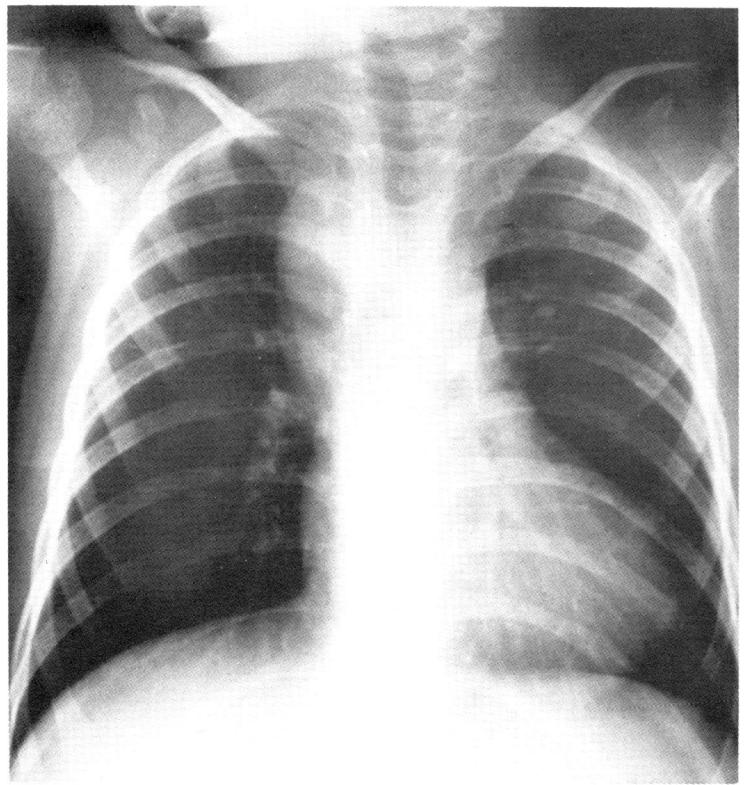

Figure 32

The abnormal features shown on this radiograph are: Right-sided Aortic Arch, an Elevated Cardiac Apex, Small Central Pulmonary Arteries, Oligaemic Lung Fields.

These features are most commonly found in Fallot's Tetralogy (in which approximately 25 per cent cases will develop this classic 'coeuren-sabot' appearance). An identical appearance can occur in Pulmonary Atresia and both conditions have a strong association with a right aortic arch (25 per cent in Fallot's tetralogy, 30–40 per cent in pulmonary atresia). The diagnosis of Fallot's Tetralogy (the diagnosis in this case) is confirmed by echocardiography but this is one of the congenital heart diseases where angiocardiography is still very important. The infundibular pulmonary stenosis, which is one of the diagnostic features, may be associated with pulmonary valve stenosis and hypoplasia of the central and peripheral pulmonary arteries. This is not well shown by echocardiography and needs to be assessed prior to surgical correction. Angiography is also required to demonstrate the bronchopulmonary and other systemic collateral arteries which are associated with severe pulmonary obstruction and the coronary artery variations which occur in about 5 per cent of cases. This information is not thought to be essential in all cases but it does make planning surgery easier and potentially less hazardous.

Case 33

This young child presented with failure to thrive, poor feeding and tachypnoea but was not cyanosed. The chest radiograph is shown in *Fig. 33a*. What abnormalities does it show and what is the differential diagnosis? How would you confirm the diagnosis?

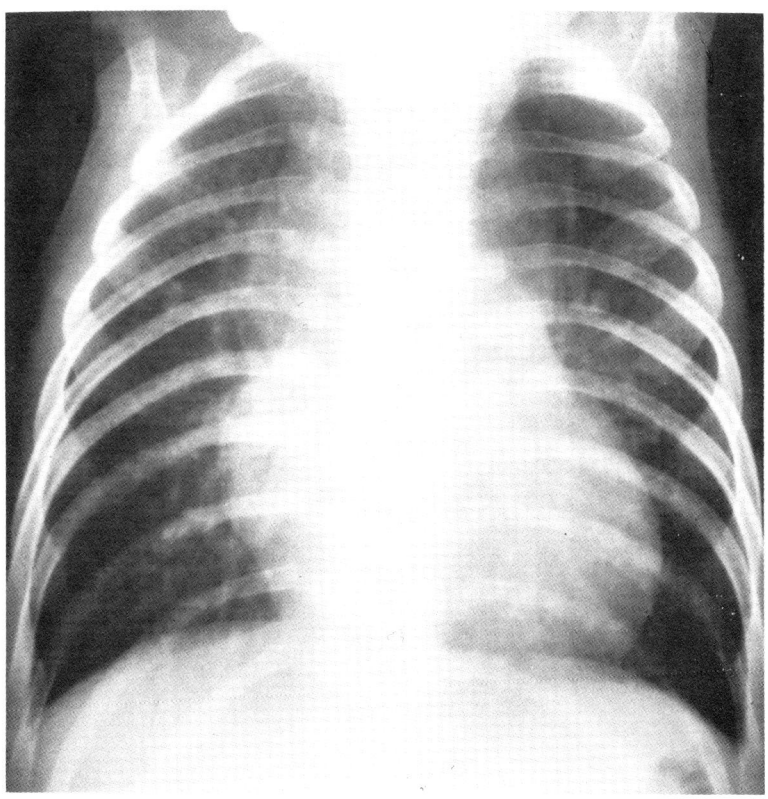

Figure 33a

The heart is enlarged and there is pulmonary plethora. The aortic arch is left sided. There are only two clear abnormalities on the radiograph but the differential diagnosis in a child who is not cyanosed and who has not had surgery is quite short. The commoner possible diagnoses are Patent Ductus Arteriosus (PDA), Ventricular Septal Defect (VSD), Atrioventricular Canal Defect and Atrial Septal Defect (ASD). Usually it is not possible to differentiate between these on the chest radiograph in children, especially at this age. There may be filling in of the normal aortopulmonary angle in patients with PDA but this is often only apparent in retrospect (as in this case which was shown to be a PDA on angiography, *Fig.* 33 *b.*

The diagnosis is confirmed by echocardiography which shows a communication between the main pulmonary artery and the descending aorta. Doppler will show continuous turbulent flow in the pulmonary artery. A number of other conditions are associated with PDA and may need to be excluded by echocardiography. These inlude ASD, VSD, pulmonary atresia, aortic arch interruption or coarctation and hypoplastic left heart syndrome.

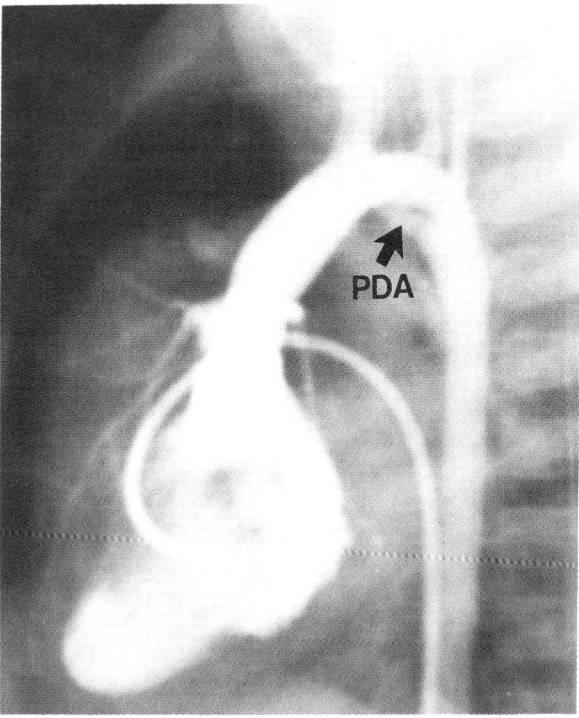

Figure 33 *b*

Case 34

This patient was admitted with a short history of severe back and abdominal pain. What is this investigation and what does it show? What other part of the body should also be examined? What alternative, and possibly better, methods of examination would be appropriate?

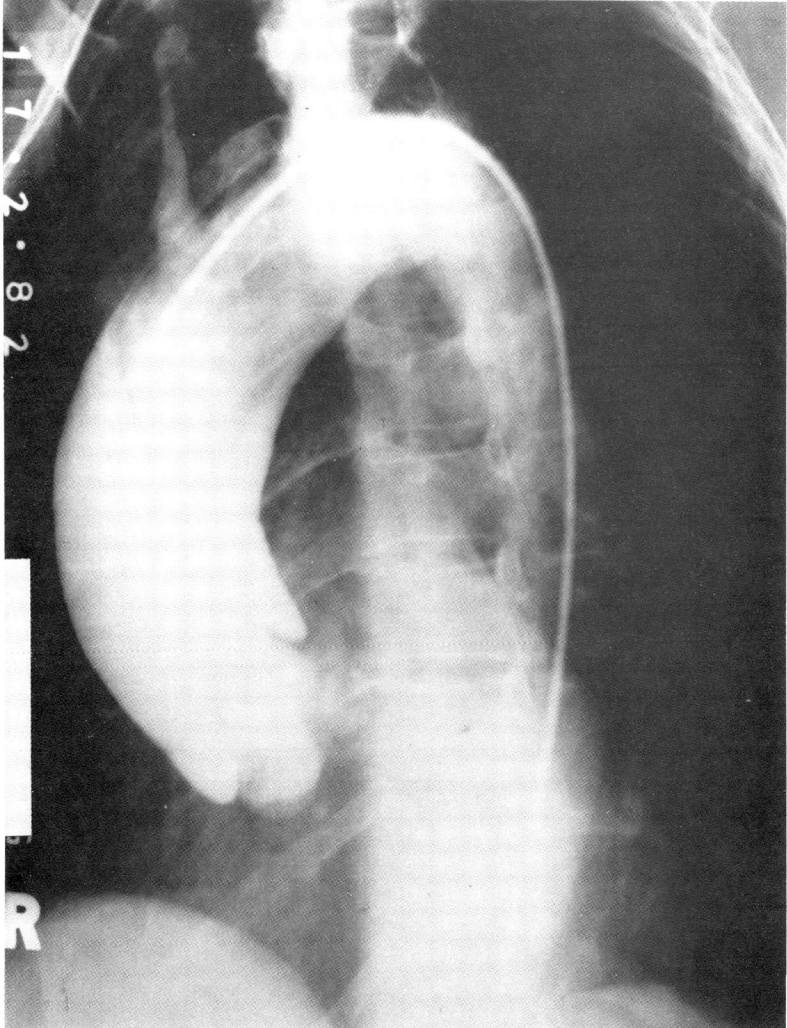

Figure 34a

This is an Arch Aortogram which shows a dissection flap in the ascending aorta which starts close to the left coronary cusp and passes vertically towards the arch of the aorta. There is poor filling of the right brachiocephalic artery. There is no aortic regurgitation. The lower extent of the dissection is not clear but in view of the history an Abdominal Aortogram is also required (*Fig.* 34*b*). The abdominal aortogram showed that there was no filling of either the superior mesenteric artery or of the right renal artery, indicating that they have been occluded by the dissection extending down to this level.

Computed tomography (CT) is usually a more reliable method of demonstrating an aortic dissection. Angiography usually requires injections in at least two projections, may be radiographically difficult and can miss a significant proportion of dissections. MRI will probably replace CT in those centres where it is available (see discussion in Case 21).

Ultrasound is valuable in establishing the diagnosis in proximal dissections and demonstrating complications such as pericardial effusions and aortic regurgitation. However, it is difficult to show the full extent of the dissection unless it extends to the abdominal aorta. Dissections which do not involve either the aortic root or the abdominal aorta are likely to be completely missed by ultrasound.

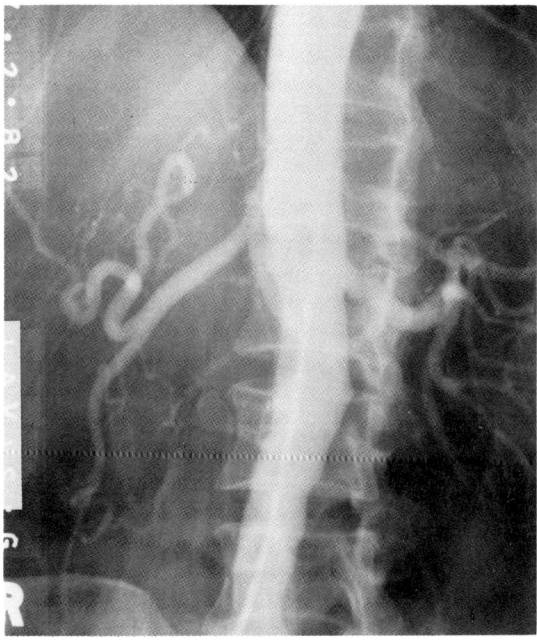

Figure 34*b*

CARDIOVASCULAR SYSTEM

Case 35

This elderly female patient is short of breath on exertion. She has been seen regularly for this in the outpatient department for many years. What does the chest radiograph show and what is the likely diagnosis? What investigation would you do next to provide the maximum useful information?

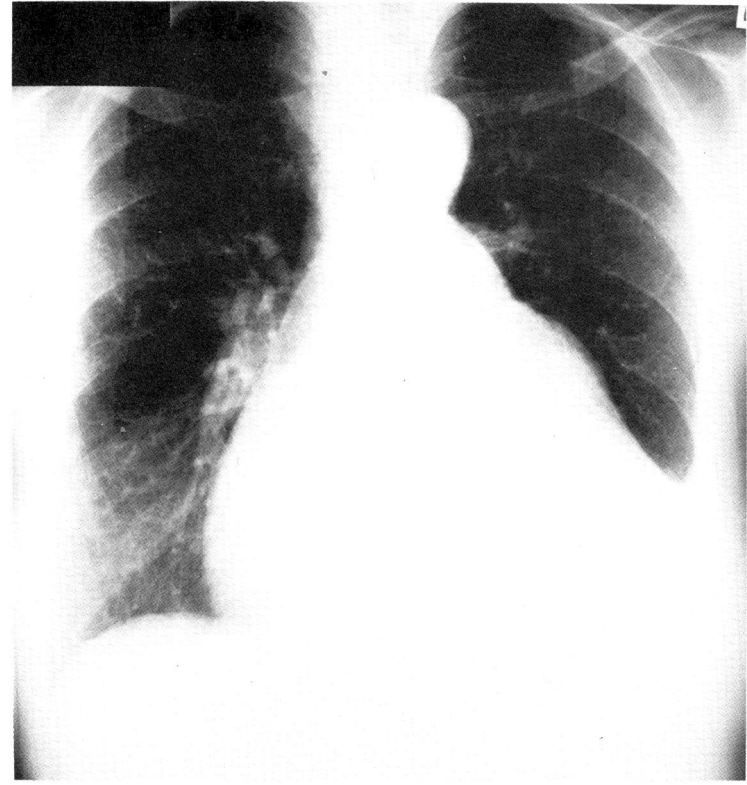

Figure 35

The cardiac shadow is considerably enlarged and is obscuring the left costophrenic angle, where there is also probably a pleural effusion. The left atrial appendage is large as is the main pulmonary artery. The left pulmonary artery is invisible on this film and the right pulmonary artery is small and the peripheral pulmonary arteries are also small. The cardiac outline suggests that this patient has Chronic Mitral Valve Disease with significant Mitral Regurgitation (indicated by the cardiomegaly). The large main pulmonary artery and small peripheral pulmonary arteries indicate that this has been complicated by the development of Pulmonary Arterial Hypertension.

The next useful examination is echocardiography, including Doppler. This will indicate the severity of the mitral regurgitation, estimate the mitral valve area and assess left ventricular function (see discussion of Cases 4 and 20). Echocardiography will also show any left atrial thrombus and detect any coexisting aortic valve disease. In the presence of pulmonary arterial hypertension there is often a degree of tricuspid regurgitation and pulmonary regurgitation. Using Doppler to measure the systolic gradient across the tricuspid valve (and to exclude pulmonary stenosis) gives a useful estimate of the severity of the pulmonary arterial hypertension.

Case 36

This investigation was performed on a 6-year-old girl. What is the investigation and what does it show? What important conditions are associated with this abnormality? What abnormality is the chest radiograph likely to show in this patient.

What alternative methods of investigation are available for demonstrating this condition?

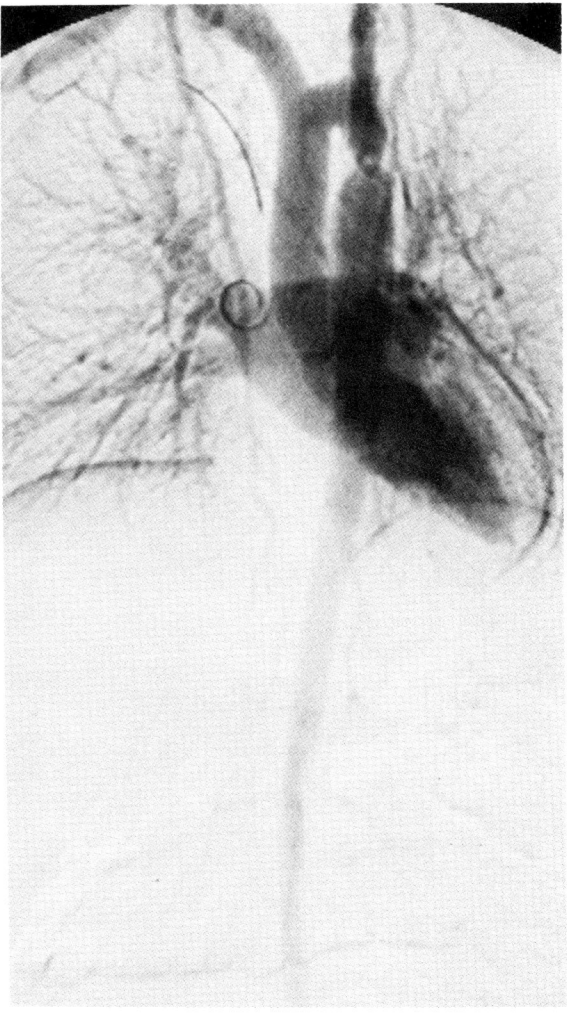

Figure 36

This is i.v. DSA Aortogram (note the pigtail catheter in the right atrium) which shows a concentric narrowing distal to the origin of the left subclavian artery. There are large internal mammary arteries but no other visible hypertrophied chest wall collaterals. This is the appearance of Coarctation of the Aorta. The patient was hypertensive and a later frame from this sequence showed the renal arteries well enough to exclude renal artery stenosis. The chest radiograph was normal, as is often the case in patients under the age of ten, in spite of a significant gradient across the coarctation. Rib notching by chest wall collaterals usually does not become apparent until after the age of ten years.

Conditions associated with coarctation of the aorta include:
1. Bicuspid aortic valve (in up to 85 per cent cases).
2. Ascending aortic aneurysm.
3. Aortic dissection.
4. Patent ductus arteriosus.
5. Aortic regurgitation.
6. Intracranial aneurysms.

Patients have hypertension proximal to the coarctation and are at increased risk of cerebrovascular disease, premature coronary artery disease and bacterial endocarditis.

Alternative imaging methods include Conventional Angiography, Echocardiography, with Doppler, and MRI. The role of clinical examination with measurement of the blood pressure in the arm and the leg is also important and often seems to be forgotten.

Case 37

What abnormalities does this radiograph show? What is the differential diagnosis of this radiographic appearance? What clinical features might help in reaching a diagnosis?

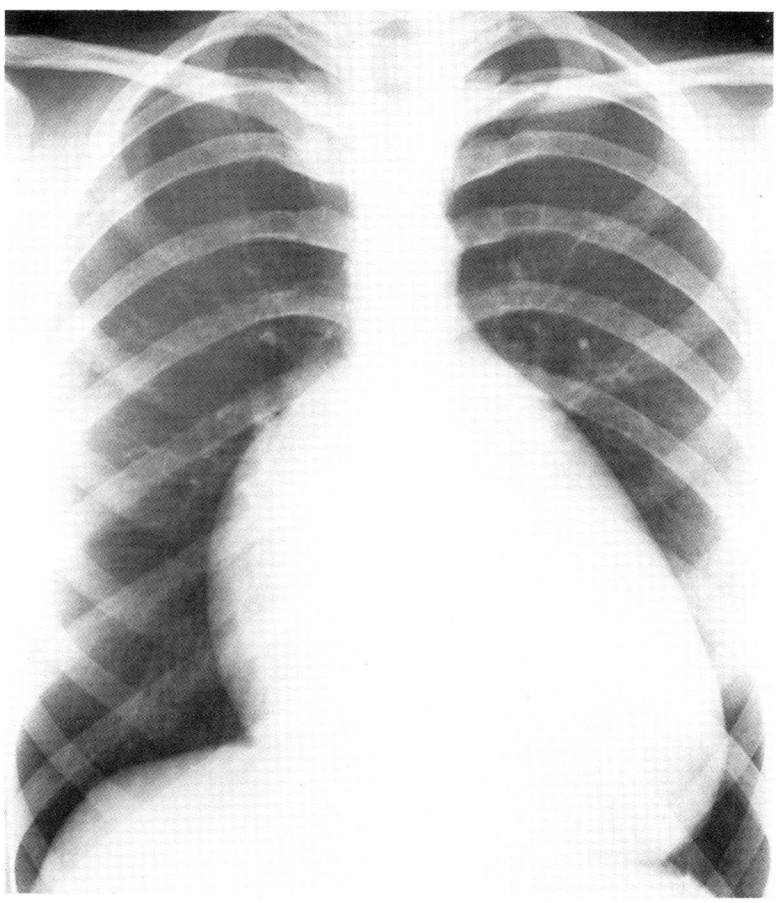

Figure 37

This chest radiograph shows a large, very well-defined cardiac shadow, small central and peripheral pulmonary vessels, a narrow vascular pedicle and a prominent smooth right heart border (suggesting right atrial enlargement). This is the characteristic chest radiographic appearance of Ebstein's Anomaly. A large well-defined heart shadow occurs when the heart is dilated and contracts poorly for whatever reason. In patients with extensive ischaemic damage, congestive cardiomyopathy or multiple valve disease there is usually a degree of pulmonary venous congestion and the pulmonary arteries are of normal size or are enlarged. Even if there has been very vigorous treatment with diuretics the pulmonary vessels should not be this small. The small pulmonary vessels suggest that there is poor forward right ventricular output. With this cardiac outline this could also be a pericardial effusion (falling blood pressure, tachycardia, abnormal venous pressure waveform), Ebstein's anomaly (stable blood pressure and central cyanosis) or Uhl's anomaly (signs may be the same as Ebstein's but this condition is very rare).

In Ebstein's anomaly there is deformity of the tricuspid valve which is displaced into the right ventricle. The combination of tricuspid regurgitation, small right ventricle and poor right ventricular contraction lead to poor pulmonary blood flow and small pulmonary vessels. There is a frequent association with right-to-left shunting across an ASD or stretched patent foramen ovale, which causes central cyanosis and this was the case in this patient.

CARDIOVASCULAR SYSTEM

Case 38

What is this investigation and what does it show? What is the significance of this finding? What complications can complicate this procedure? What alternative methods are available for investigating this sort of problem?

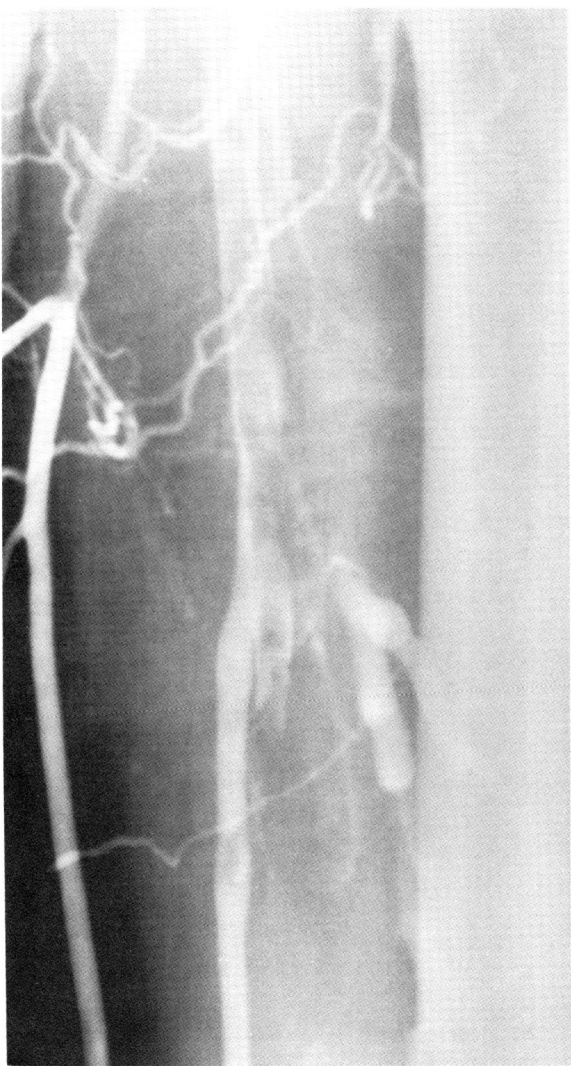

Figure 38

This is an Ascending Leg Venogram which shows thrombus in the femoral veins. The thrombus seems to arise from veins which are almost completely filled with thrombus and projects into the more proximal veins. The thrombus may be more extensive than is apparent on this view being present in parts of the veins which have not been filled as they are completely filled with thrombus. It is generally thought that thrombus limited to the calf veins is less likely to cause significant pulmonary embolization than thrombus in the larger proximal veins of the thigh and the pelvis.

Ascending venography can be a difficult procedure to perform and can be very Painful, even with the use of non-ionic contrast media. There is also a risk, albeit a small one, of Dislodging Thrombus and causing a Pulmonary Embolus. In patients who have had a large pulmonary embolus the administration of contrast media can cause a significant drop in Cardiac Output with Hypotension which can lead to Syncope. Other complications include Chemical Phlebitis and Superficial Necrosis around the injection site, which is now uncommon with non-ionic contrast media, and contrast medium related reactions. These complications have led to the development of alternative methods for diagnosing deep vein thrombosis. These methods include:
Isotope Venography
Isotope Labelled Fibrinogen Uptake
Isotope Labelled Platelet Uptake
Doppler Ultrasound
Cross-sectional Ultrasound
MRI

All of these methods have drawbacks and venography is still regarded as the most accurate method for making the diagnosis of deep vein thrombosis. There are, however, a number of situations where less invasive methods are useful. It should be noted that thermography is not included on this list as its accuracy is too poor for it to be useful in clinical practice.

Case 39

This patient was admitted as an emergency with a history of recent chest pain, which sounded like angina, and a long history of being blue and short of breath. This is his chest radiograph taken on admission. What does it show? What is the underlying condition which is responsible for this appearance, for his cyanosis and for his breathlessness?

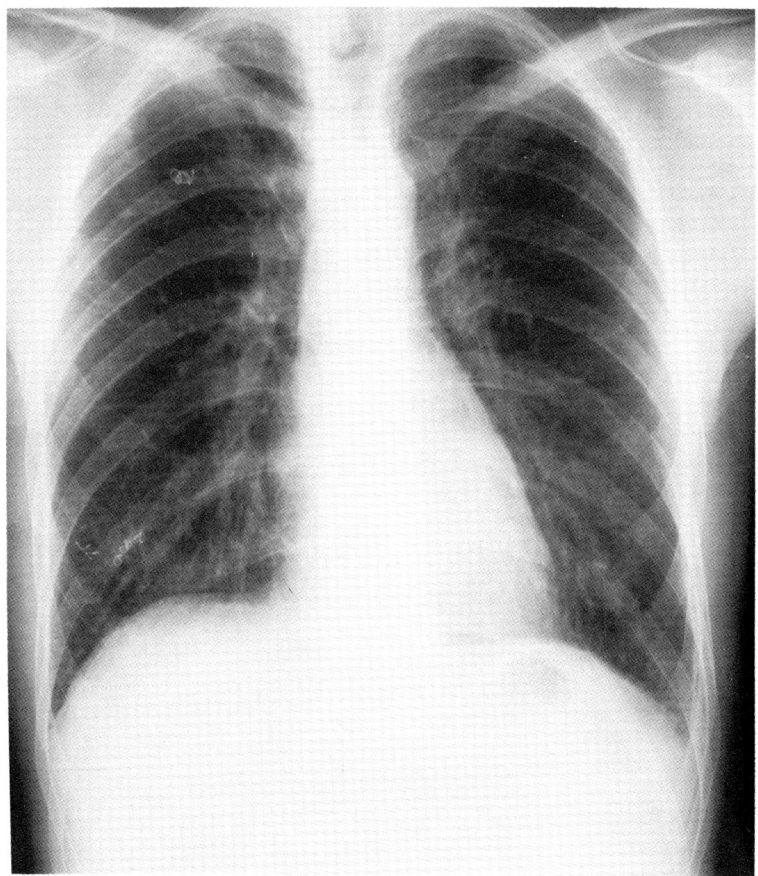

Figure 39

The chest radiograph shows a number of metallic coils in the right lung (eight in all). These are Gianturco–Wallace Coils which were used to embolize some of the Pulmonary Arteriovenous Malformations which had caused him to be cyanosed for many years. The rest of the chest radiograph is unremarkable.

Arteriovenous malformations can occur anywhere in the body and are often very difficult to treat surgically. In the lungs they are usually best treated by embolization, using steel coils or silicone balloons introduced percutaneously through catheters under radiological control. In other parts of the body other embolization materials such as glue, alcohol, dura mater, hyperosmolar dextrose, gelatin sponge and blood clot may be used. As an increasing number of patients are treated in this way the radiopaque devices will be more commonly seen on radiographs. Embolization using these and other materials is also used to treat an assortment of other conditions including tumours and haemorrhage due to a variety of local conditions.

Pulmonary arteriovenous malformations can cause a variety of symptoms due to hypoxia, polycythaemia and systemic embolization. Most of those malformations which can be treated by embolization should be treated in this way. Embolization is very effective in improving oxygenation by reducing arteriovenous shunting, and therefore reducing polycythaemia. Therapeutic embolization is also very successful in reducing the risks of systemic embolization and this is an important reason for recommending treatment, preferably before systemic embolization (causing stroke, renal infarction, etc.) has occurred.

Case 40

What abnormality does this echocardiogram show? What specific areas should be examined in this patient? What is the differential diagnosis?

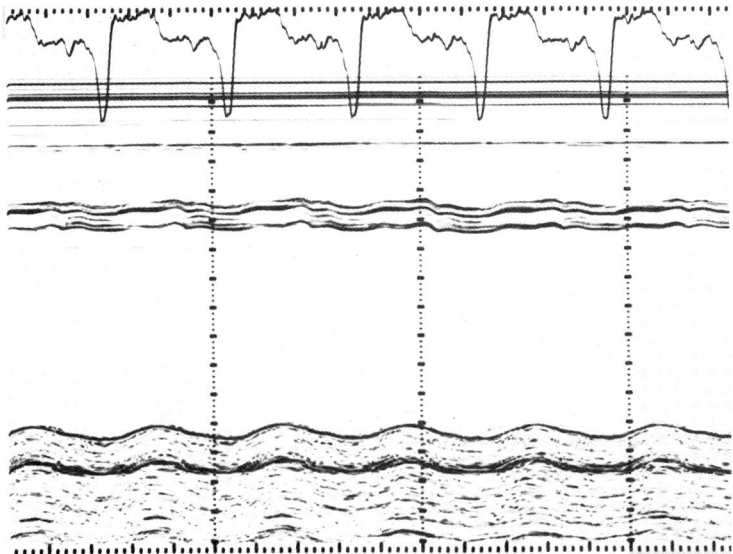

Figure 40a

This M-mode Echocardiogram shows a dilated, poorly contracting left ventricle (compare with the normal tracing shown in *Fig.* 40*b*). The end-diastolic diameter is 7 cm and the end-systolic diameter is 6·7 cm giving a calculated ejection fraction of 12·5 per cent. The walls of the ventricle are not thickened. The ECG which is also displayed shows a bundle branch type pattern. These are the features of severe, generalized left ventricular dysfunction which occurs most commonly in Congestive Cardiomyopathy, where cardiomyopathy is used in the broadest sense of the word to describe generalized heart muscle disease. A similar appearance can occur in patients with widespread ischaemic heart disease, although the pattern of impaired ventricular contraction may be irregular in cases of ischaemic heart disease, and in patients with longstanding severe mitral regurgitation or aortic valve disease (stenosis or regurgitation).

Specific attention should be given to the presence of intraventricular trombus, the degree of mitral regurgitation and the aortic valve, to exclude end-stage aortic stenosis or regurgitation. The diagnosis in this case was aortic stenosis.

The further differential diagnosis of the causes of this type of generalized heart muscle disease is large but the important causes in the United Kingdom include: Congestive Cardiomyopathy (Idiopathic), Myocarditis (including viral and toxic), Chronic Hypertensive Heart Disease, Chronic Alcoholic Heart Disease, Cytotoxic Drugs, Familial Neuromuscular syndromes, Endocardial Fibroelastosis, Haemochromatosis.

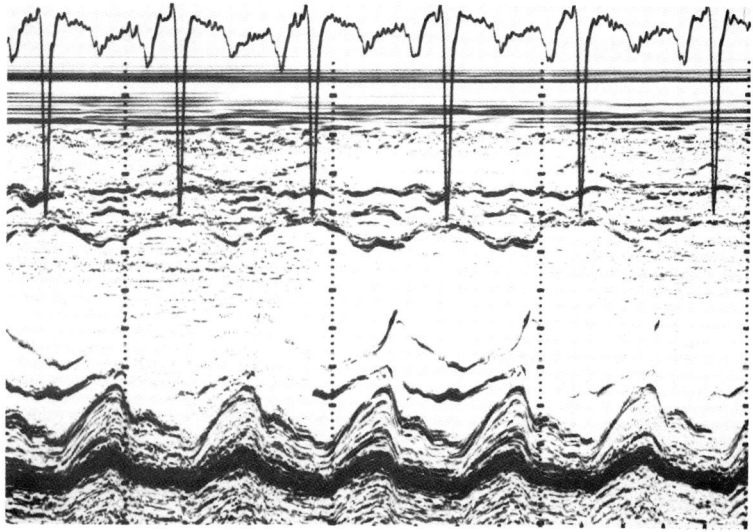

Figure 40*b*

Case 41

This examination was performed on a 26-year-old woman. What is the examination and what does it show? What further radiographic information is required to allow full interpretation of this examination? What is the likely diagnosis and what possible alternatives are there?

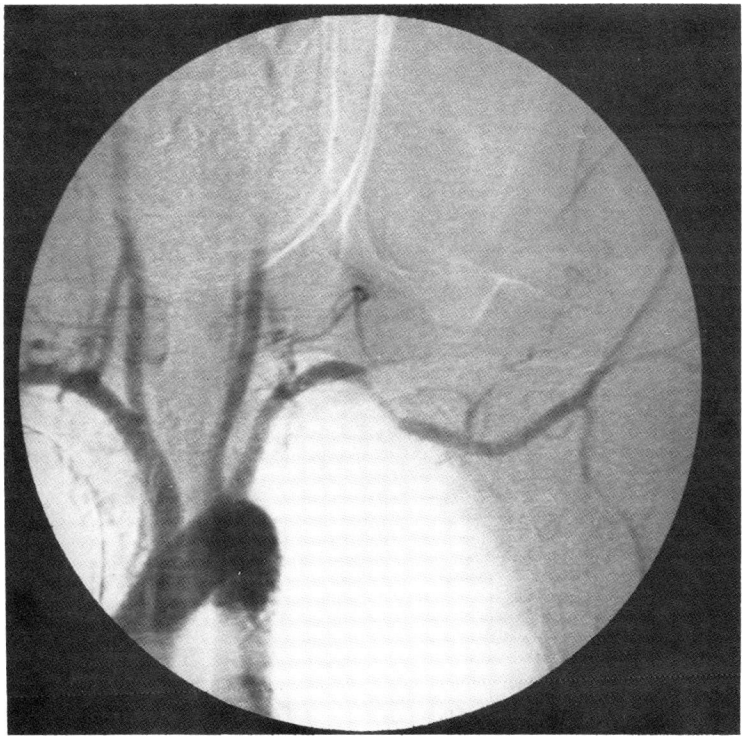

Figure 41*a*

This is an Intravenous DSA Subclavian Arteriogram taken with the patient's arm abducted (note the orientation of the axillary artery) which shows a short eccentric narrowing of the subclavian artery as it passes behind the left clavicle. The artery on either side of this narrow segment looks normal as do the other arteries visible on this image. Further interpretation is only possible if it is known whether this is a constant feature or if it is position dependent. *Fig.* 41 *b* is the control angiogram from this patient with the arm adducted and shows that in this position the left subclavian artery appears normal. This indicates that there is position-dependent compression and in a patient of this age compression by a Cervical Band is the most likely diagnosis. A plain radiograph should be examined for evidence of a Cervical Rib, although this is less likely to cause compression alone.

Other alternative diagnoses for the initial image include compression by local masses (such as tumour), stricturing following local trauma (such as shoulder girdle injury and during central venous cannulation) or dissection by catheters introduced from the brachial artery.

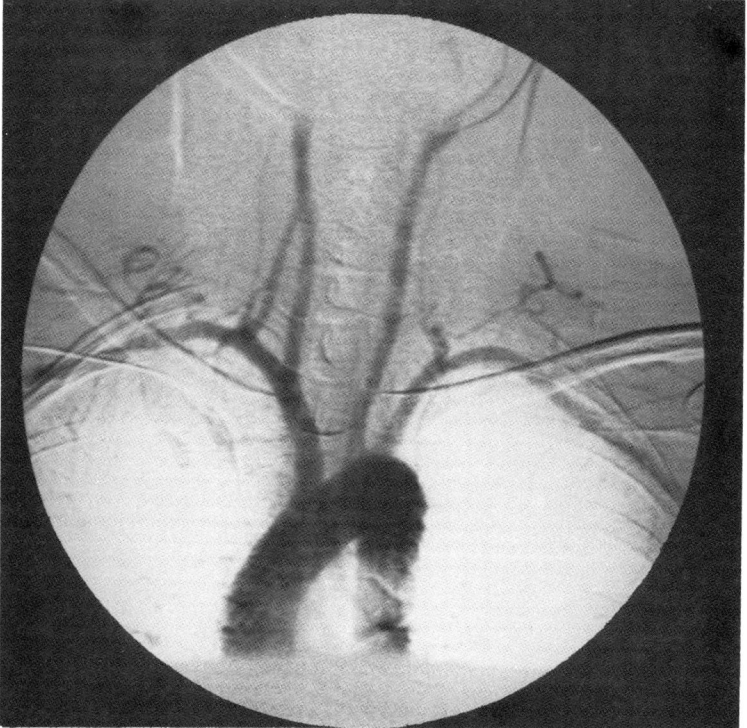

Figure 41 *b*

CARDIOVASCULAR SYSTEM 83

Case 42

This is a contrast enhanced CT scan from a 65-year-old man with a vague abdominal pain. What does it show and what is the significance of these findings? What further information is required from this investigation?

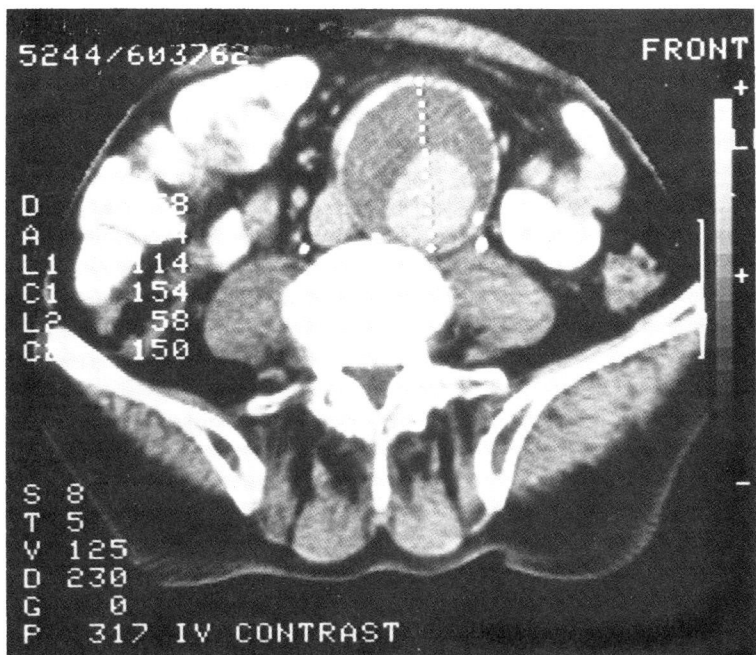

Figure 42

There is a large abdominal aortic aneurysm which contains extensive thrombus. The aneurysm is well defined by a rim of calcification with no evidence of a surrounding soft-tissue mass or haematoma around most of its circumference. However, there is a small high attenuation area adjacent to it (at 10'o'clock) but outside the line of the calcified wall. The ureters are separate from it and are not dilated at this level. The presence of a large abdominal aortic aneurysm, even in an asymptomatic patient, suggests that there is an increased risk of aortic rupture and this becomes increasingly likely as the overall diameter of the aneurysm increases. This is particularly so when the diameter rises above 5 cm (the diameter in this case is shown to be 5·8 cm). The presence of an enhancing soft-tissue mass of this type, even if the mass is small, outside the line of the calcified wall of the aneurysm indicates that this is an inflammatory aneurysm. Inflammatory aneurysms have a worse prognosis than ordinary atheromatous aneurysms but are more difficult to treat surgically and are associated with an increased surgical mortality and morbidity. The separation of the ureters from the aneurysm makes surgery easier and should be positively commented on. The presence of the extensive clot is probably of little significance.

The other important points which should be assessed by CT include:

1. More proximal ureteric involvement and evidence of ureteric obstruction.
2. Perfusion of the kidneys.
3. To exclude other intra-abdominal abnormalities which may complicate surgery (i.e. unexpected horseshoe kidneys).
4. The upper level of the aneurysm, particularly with regard to the level of the renal arteries. To show these reliably requires careful attention to technique with close CT sections at the level of the origins of the renal arteries. Aneurysms extending to the level of the renal arteries or above may require a more extensive (thoraco-abdominal) approach than aneurysms which start more distally. In difficult cases angiography may be required to show the renal arteries.

Case 43

What is this investigation and what does it show? What are the conditions which may be associated with this appearance? What are the therapeutic implications? What are the plain radiograph appearances? What other investigations may be useful?

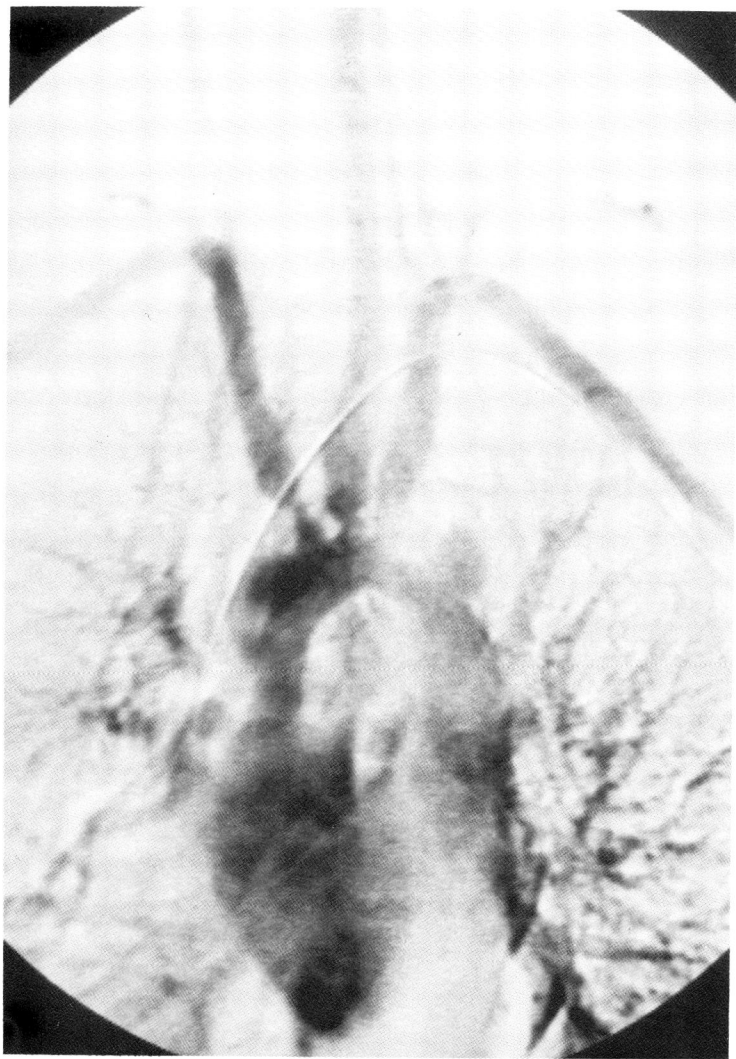

Figure 43

This is an Intravenous DSA Arch Aortogram (note the venous catheter passing from the left arm to the right atrium). There is a short area of Supravalvar Aortic Stenosis with an area of post-stenotic dilatation. There is narrowing of the origins of the neck vessels and the right common carotid artery is occluded at its origin. There is a Saccular Aneurysm of the distal aortic arch (which followed surgical repair of a severe coarctation at this site). Supravalvar Aortic Stenosis is often associated with the syndrome of Infantile Hypercalcaemia (associated with Mental Deficiency, Abnormal facies, Peripheral Pulmonary Artery Stenosis).

Initially if there is significant stenosis there is left ventricular strain and surgical repair is required to prevent deterioration in ventricular function. There may be more distal areas of narrowing in the aorta (as in this case where there was a discrete coarctation requiring repair) and the major aortic branches. In this case the origins of the left subclavian, left common carotid and brachiocephalic arteries are narrowed and the origin of the right common carotid artery is totally occluded. When the stenosing process is this extensive surgical repair is very difficult.

The plain radiographic features are non-specific. The left ventricle is enlarged but the ascending aorta is usually small, unlike patients with valvar aortic stenosis. The left atrium may be enlarged and there may be evidence of pulmonary venous congestion resulting from the high filling pressures required to fill the hypertrophied left ventricle.

The area of the supravalvar stenosis may be visible on echocardiography and Doppler can give an estimate of the severity of the gradient across the stenotic area. Duplex Doppler may be valuable in assessing the degree of involvement of the carotid and subclavian arteries.

Full cardiac catheterization with pressure measurements and imaging of the coronary arteries (by aortography in children, selective angiography in adults) is required before surgery.

Case 44

This is the chest radiograph of a patient admitted for investigation of worsening ill health over a period of several weeks. His symptoms included fever and peripheral swelling. What does the chest radiograph show? What are the possible differential diagnoses and which of these is the most likely in this case? What are the causes of this condition and what is the most appropriate confirmatory investigation?

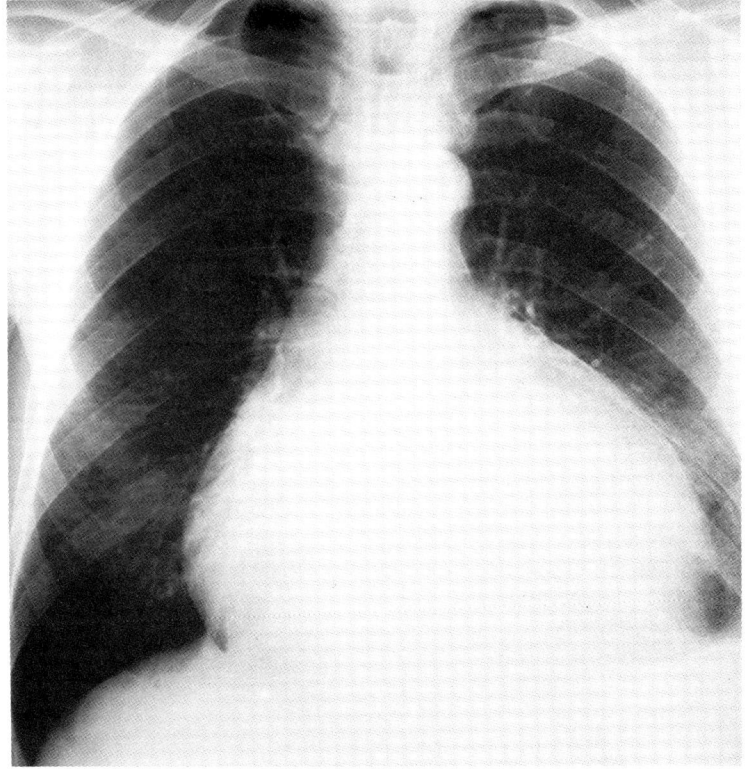

Figure 44

This chest radiograph shows marked enlargement of the cardiac shadow but normal lung fields. There is no evidence of abnormal calcification and the shape of the cardiac shadow is globular and well defined. The possible causes of this type of globular enlargement include Multiple Valve Disease, Diffuse Heart Muscle Disease (whatever the aetiology), Ebstein's Anomaly and Pericardial Effusion. In the presence of normal lung fields the first two diagnoses are relatively unlikely, although patients treated with large doses of diuretics may have normal pulmonary vessels. Ebstein's anomaly (see Case 37) is uncommon, usually does not look quite like this and is not consistent with the short history. The likeliest diagnosis radiographically, particularly in this context, is pericardial effusion.

In this patient who had recently returned from an area where tuberculosis is common the diagnosis was tuberculous pericarditis with a large pericardial effusion. In tuberculous pericarditis the effusion can become very large without causing much haemodynamic deterioration.

Echocardiography is usually the most appropriate confirmatory investigation (see Case 29). Pericardial Aspiration may be required to make a bacteriological or cytological diagnosis.

Other important causes of pericardial effusion include:
1. Infective Pericarditis due to Viral Infection or Pyogenic Organisms.
2. Dressler's Syndrome following myocardial infarction or cardiac surgery.
3. Connective Tissue Disorders, particularly Rheumatoid Arthritis, Systemic Lupus Erythematosus and Scleroderma.
4. Malignancy, which can result from direct invasion by local tumour (Carcinoma Bronchus, Mesothelioma), Metastases and Lymphoma.
5. Aortic Dissection.
6. Heart Failure.
7. Myxoedema.
8. Uraemia.
9. Chest Trauma.

CARDIOVASCULAR SYSTEM

Case 45

What abnormality is shown on this M-mode echocardiogram? What further investigations are required?

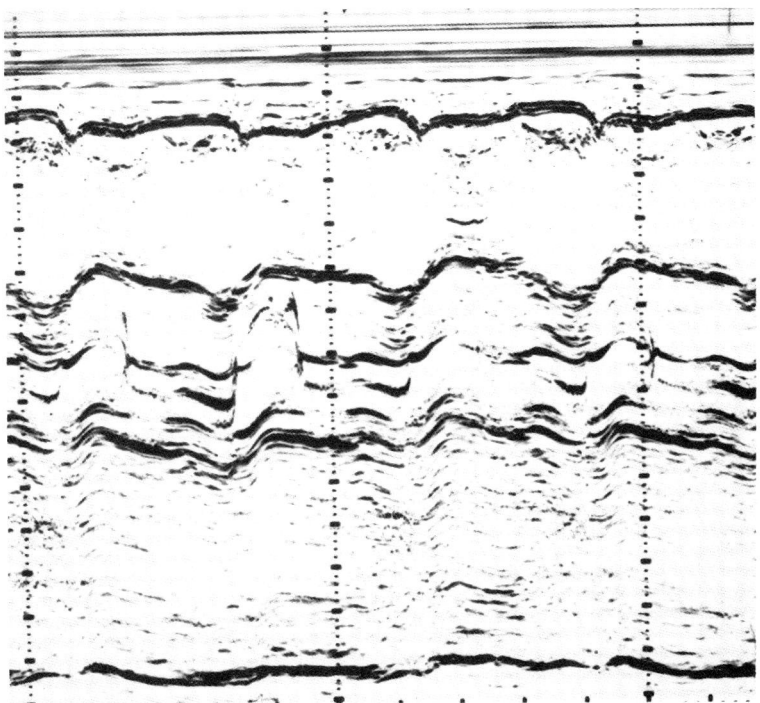

Figure 45 a

This M-mode echocardiogram shows abnormal echoes in the aortic root, seen best during diastole, although the aortic valve cusps are mobile and are not thickened. The diameter of the left atrium is apparently increase (5 cm). The aortic valve appearances are due to Vegetations on the valve in this patient with Bacterial Endocarditis. This should be confirmed by 2-D echocardiography (*Figure* 45*b* which shows the echodense vegetations on the aortic valve (←) and also shows that the left atrium (LA) is not enlarged). Echocardiography alone does not make the diagnosis of endocarditis, similar appearances can sometimes be produced by valve calcification, valve prolapse and small prominences on the valve cusps. The diagnosis should be confirmed by the appropriate bacteriological and immunological methods. In the appropriate clinical circumstances, especially if there is Doppler evidence of valve regurgitation, the echocardiogram is helpful in suggesting the diagnosis before bacteriological results are available and allowing treatment to start early. Echocardiography is also valuable in assessing any change in murmurs or haemodynamics and demonstrating complications such as abscess formation.

It should be remembered that vegetations can persist for long periods after bacteriological cure and therefore echocardiography is of limited value in monitoring these patients unless there is clinical evidence of deterioration.

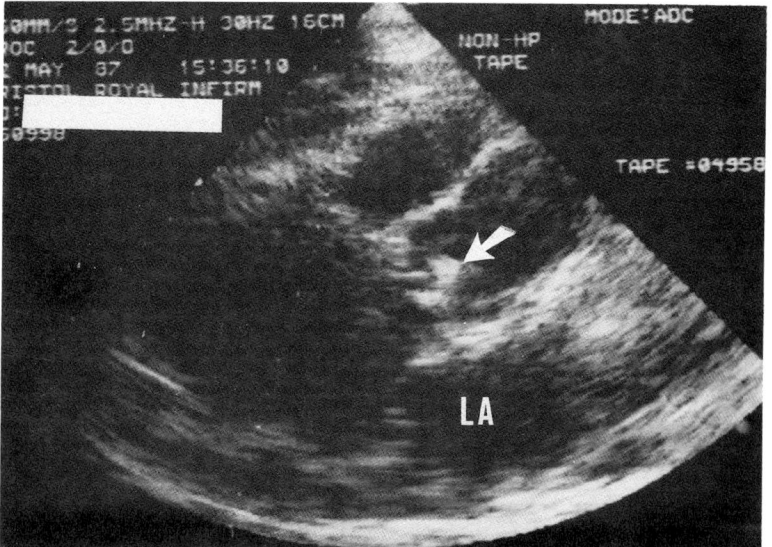

Figure 45*b*

Case 46

What is this investigation and what does it show? Would you perform it this way? This patient is very ill as a result of the abnormality seen here. What would you do next?

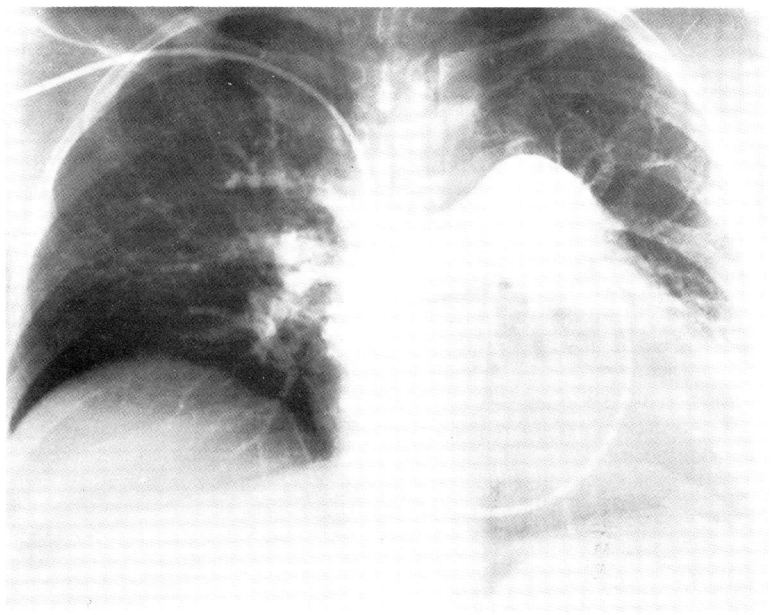

Figure 46

This is a Pulmonary Arteriogram which shows clot in the right upper and lower lobe pulmonary arteries. There is patchy underperfusion of both lungs, although clot is not clearly seen on the left as the pulmonary arteries on that side are obscured by the density of the heart. In this case an injection has been made into the main pulmonary artery and the whole of the chest is shown on a single film. Although this showed the clot, in this case a very large injection of contrast medium was required to achieve satisfactory opacification of the pulmonary arteries. In sick patients with severe pulmonary artery obstruction by clot, as in this case, the haemodynamic effects of a large injection can cause a further catastrophic reduction in blood pressure. Selective injections into the lobar pulmonary arteries are usually now used as smaller volumes are used for each injection and cause less haemodynamic deterioration. Also smaller fields of view using oblique (and preferably bi-plane) projections show clot more clearly, especially behind the heart and at the bases of the lung where the diaphragms may obscure abnormalities.

Having established the diagnosis of pulmonary embolism and showing that the emboli are too peripheral for surgical removal the next step is to infuse streptokinase through the angiographic catheter to dissolve the clot. Fortunately the catheter has been introduced from an arm vein, which is a much more convenient position for patient management than a femoral catheter and is probably safer, with a lower risk of unnoticed haematoma formation around the puncture site.

Case 47

This patient was admitted to the Coronary Care Unit after an extensive inferior myocardial infarction for which he required a temporary pacemaker. What abnormalities does this chest radiograph show?

List six complications of pacing (permanent or temporary) which can be demonstrated on a chest radiograph.

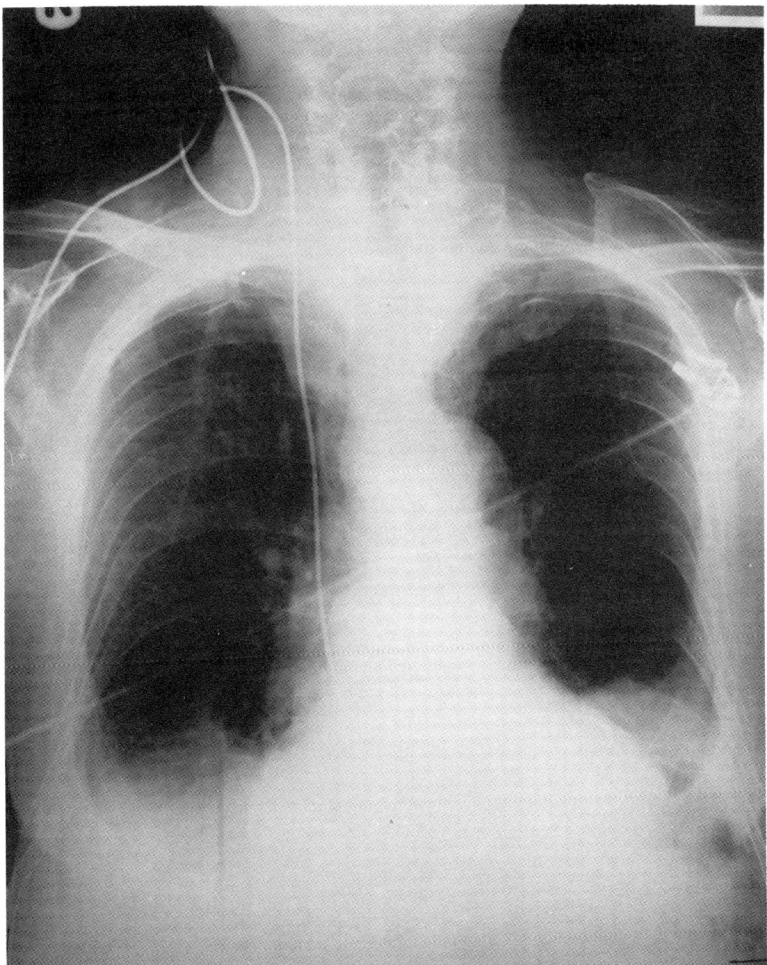

Figure 47

This is an AP chest radiograph, as can be seen from the position of the scapulae, ribs and the orientation of the cervical spinous processes. Therefore it is difficult to assess cardiac size accurately but in this case it may be normal. The abnormalities seen are:
1. Perforation of the Myocardium by the Pacing Wire (the tip of which can be seen curved around the left heart border).
2. Bilateral Pleural Effusions.
3. Soft-tissue swelling at the base of the neck due to Haematoma following multiple attempts at jugular vein puncture.
4. Widening of the Superior Mediastinum with a right apical cap due to Pleural Haematoma (in this case associated with erroneous subclavian artery puncture).
Careful examination of the lung fields shows that there is no pneumothorax.
Other complications of pacing visible on a chest radiograph include:
1. Pacing wire fractures (now relatively uncommon).
2. Pneumothorax.
3. Pericardial Effusion from myocardial perforation leading to haemopericardium and possibly tamponade.
4. Surgical emphysema.
5. Knots in the pacing wire.
6. Malposition of the pacing wire tip (reported sites include coronary sinus, hepatic veins, left ventricle, coronary artery, cardiac veins, pericardium).
7. Migration of the pacing wire from its intended site (back into right atrium, IVC, SVC, pulmonary artery).
8. Generator migration and lead twisting (Twiddler's syndrome).
9. Gas surrounding the pacemaker generator in cases of infected pacemaker pocket.

Case 48

This 2-week-old child was referred for investigation of cyanosis, poor feeding and tachypnoea. What does this chest radiograph show and what common feature can simulate this appearance? What would be your next useful investigation to establish the diagnosis?

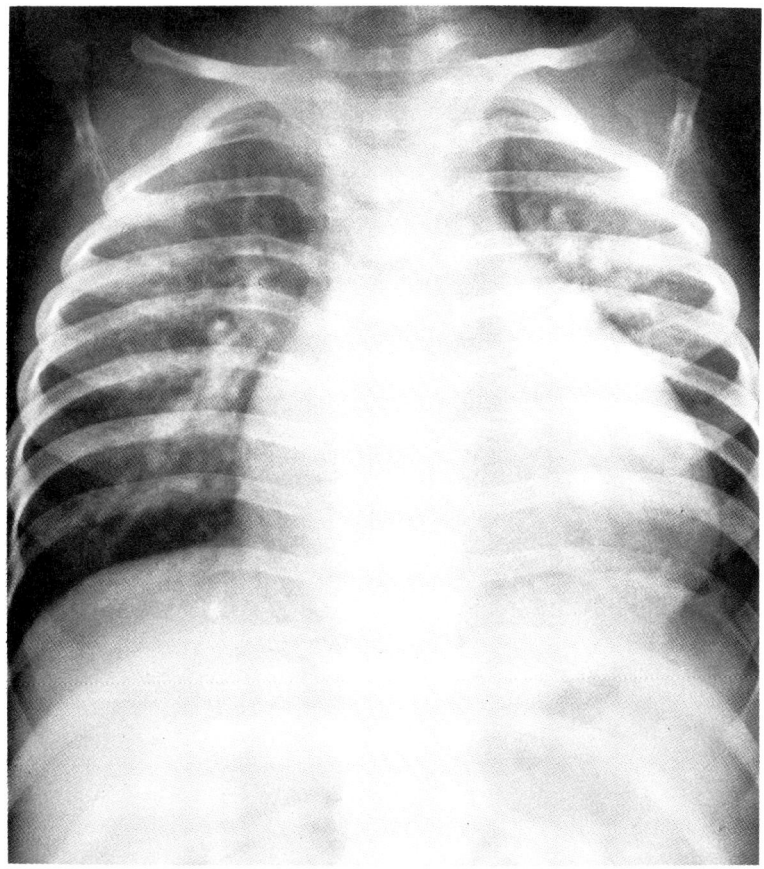

Figure 48*a*

This chest radiograph shows a normal size heart with pulmonary plethora and a widened superior mediastinum. A wide superior mediastinum at this age is often due to an enlarged thymus, but the thymus is usually denser, better defined and of a different, asymmetrical shape. The combination of a wide superior mediastinum of this configuration ('Snowman' or 'Cottage Loaf') and pulmonary plethora is one of the few characteristic chest radiograph appearances in congenital heart disease at this age. The diagnosis is Supracardiac Total Anomalous Pulmonary Venous Drainage (TAPVD), which is the commonest type of TAPVD. Infracardiac TAPVD (see Case 7) occurs in 10 per cent cases, is always associated with obstruction and presents very early with severe pulmonary venous congestion. Intracardiac TAPVD presents like the supracardiac form but with a normal superior mediastinum.

Echocardiography will confirm the diagnosis, demonstrate the associated ASD and show any obstructing septa or kinking of the anomalous veins. If further anatomical information is required angiography, with an injection into the anomalous vein or during the venous phase following a pulmonary artery injection (*Fig.* 48*b*), shows the anatomy very well.

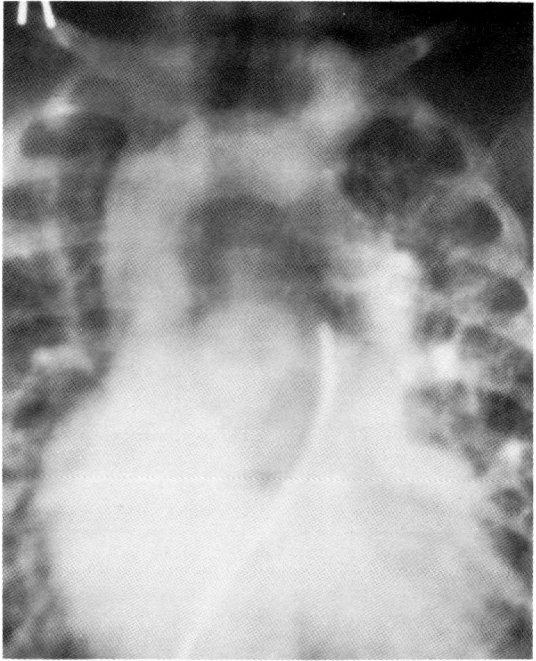

Figure 48*b*

Case 49

What abnormalities are shown on this chest radiograph of a 2-year-old child? The child is mildly cyanosed. What are the possible likely diagnoses?

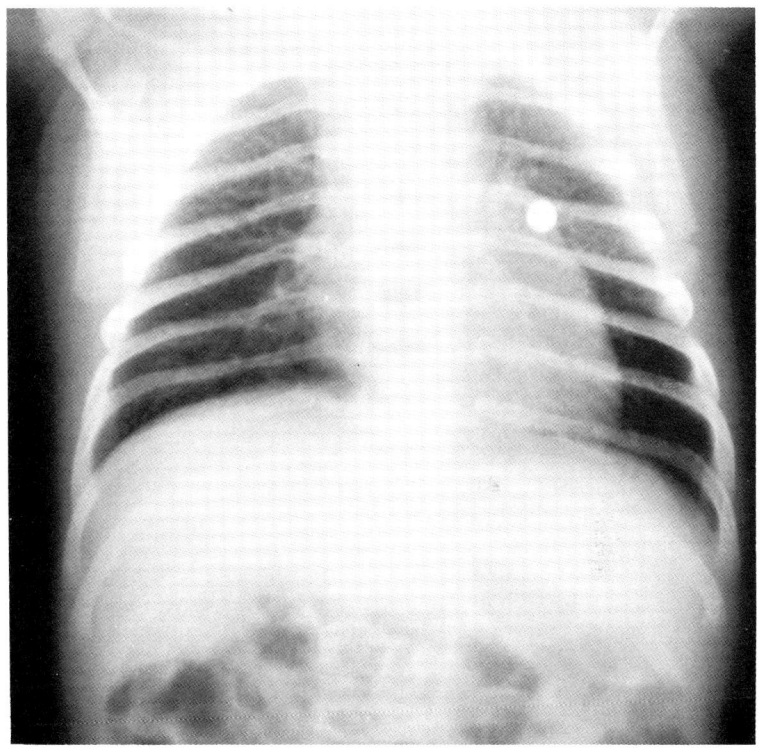

Figure 49

The liver has a horizontal inferior border and extends across the full width of the upper abdomen. The stomach is not clearly visible. The heart size is normal. The lung fields are oligaemic (this is a rather 'soft' film—look particularly at the lower lung fields). There is a right internal jugular vein cannula. The abnormal liver is the important observation in this case as it is the key to identifying this as a case of complex congenital heart disease.

The presence of this type of midline liver indicates the presence of asplenia, although polysplenia may also be associated with a midline liver and stomach. Asplenia is usually associated with Right Atrial Isomerism, which can be confirmed by echocardiography or angiography, and Right Bronchial Isomerism, which is difficult to see on neonatal chest radiographs. The normal size heart and oligaemic lung fields indicate a degree of obstruction to pulmonary flow. There are many cardiac abnormalities associated with asplenia, which is a good marker of complex severe congenital heart disease. The major associated conditions are those resulting from defects of cardiac septation and include:
1. Persistent Atrioventricular Canal.
2. Single ventricle.
3. Single atrium.
4. Total Anomalous Pulmonary Venous Drainage.
5. Atrioventricular and Ventriculo-Arterial Discordance.
6. Conotruncal abnormalities.
7. Pulmonary Atresia.

These abnormalities can occur in a variety of more or less complicated combinations; it is often impossible to assess them any further from the chest radiograph, except to comment on pulmonary perfusion. Echocardiography, and sometimes angiography, is required to make the diagnosis, as was the case in this patient who had right atrial isomerism, atrioventricular discordance, transposed great arteries, ventricular septal defect, patent ductus arteriosus and pulmonary atresia.

Case 50

This adult patient was admitted with a three-week history of intermittent fever and weight loss. He had a Starr–Edwards mitral valve replacement a year before admission. As a result of clinical examination a DSA femoral arteriogram was performed. This is shown in *Fig.* 50. What does this show? What is the likely diagnosis and what further investigations are indicated?

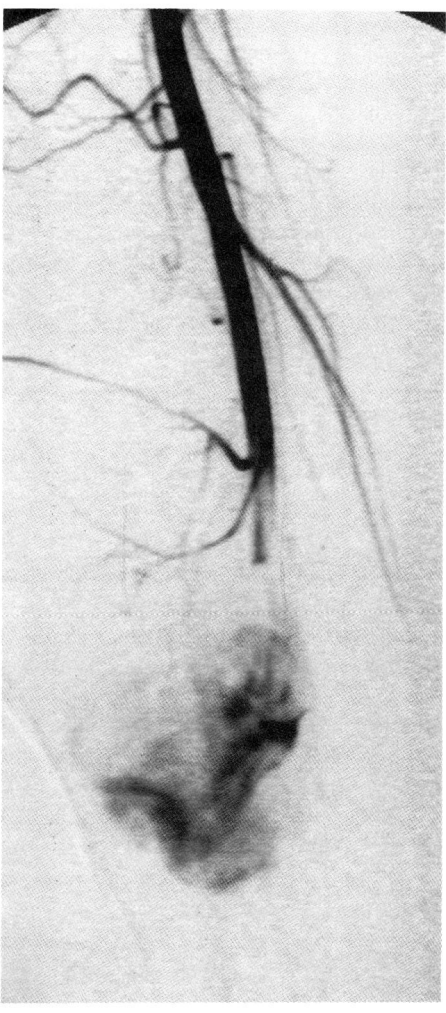

Figure 50

There is an abrupt break in the line of the popliteal artery lumen with a filling defect within it. Contrast is filling a large irregular cavity beyond the end of the vessel which must represent a pseudo-aneurysm. In the clinical context this most probably represents a Mycotic Aneurysm complicating Endocarditis on the mitral valve replacement. The filling defect in the stump of the artery may represent the Septic Embolus.

Further investigations are directed at confirming the diagnosis, e.g. by blood culture, and assessing any other complications affecting the valve prosthesis and its function. In patients with a highly echogenic ball and cage prosthesis, such as the Starr–Edwards valve, echocardiography seldom shows any structural abnormality except in gross cases or where the endocarditis has spread into the surrounding tissue to form an abscess or paravalvar fistula. However, Doppler is useful for showing evidence of valve dysfunction or paravalvar leaks which may support the diagnosis of endocarditis. CT scanning is not helpful as the metal in the valve cage causes extensive artefact around the valve which makes it impossible to get clear images of the area in question. This is less of a problem with MRI where there may be little artefact around the valve prosthesis and paravalvar abscesses not seen on CT or ultrasound may be visualized. Angiography is seldom helpful and manipulating a catheter close to valve vegetations may cause further systemic embolization.

Case 51

This elderly patient has recently become short of breath. He is being treated for carcinoma of the prostate but at his recent clinic assessment there was no evidence of active prostatic disease. What does his current chest radiograph show? What is the likely diagnosis? What further investigation would you advise?

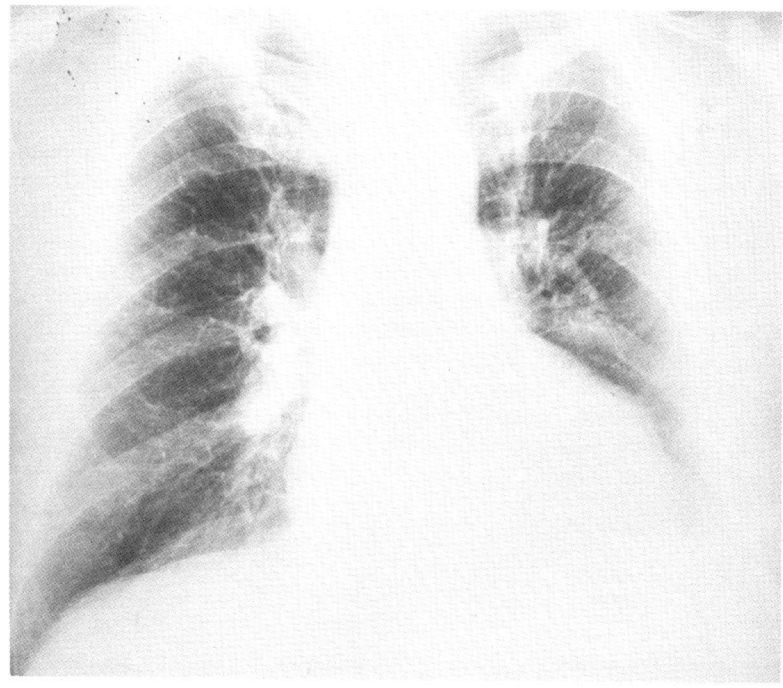

Figure 51*a*

There is an abrupt reduction in the size of the right lower lobe pulmonary artery associated with a paucity of peripheral vessels in the right lower zone. The pulmonary vessels on the left appear normal. There is no evidence of pulmonary oedema. The heart is slightly enlarged. The bones visible on this film appear normal. The features suggest a Right-sided Pulmonary Embolus and a ventilation perfusion lung scan is advised.

The abnormalities in the right lower zone are the most important diagnostic features and are therefore mentioned first. The absence of pulmonary oedema in a patient with a known carcinoma is an important negative feature as the diagnosis of lymphangitis carcinomatosa is often missed. A comment on the bones is also relevant as prostatic carcinoma disseminates to bone early in the course of the disease. The large heart in a patient with this history could be due to coexistent ischaemic heart disease, unrelated valve or hypertensive heart disease (all of which are common in this age group) or pericardial effusion (which could be due to secondary invasion by tumour or uraemia caused by chronic urinary obstruction).

The need for a ventilation perfusion lung scan (see discussions of (cases 19 and 28) is clearly indicated by the radiographic abnormalities. Although these are clear cut in this case the diagnosis of pulmonary emboli on the basis of plain film changes is unreliable. The lung scan (*Fig.* 51*b*—anterior perfusion image) showed very poor perfusion of the right lung (with almost normal ventilation seen on the ventilation scan) confirming the diagnosis of a large pulmonary embolus.

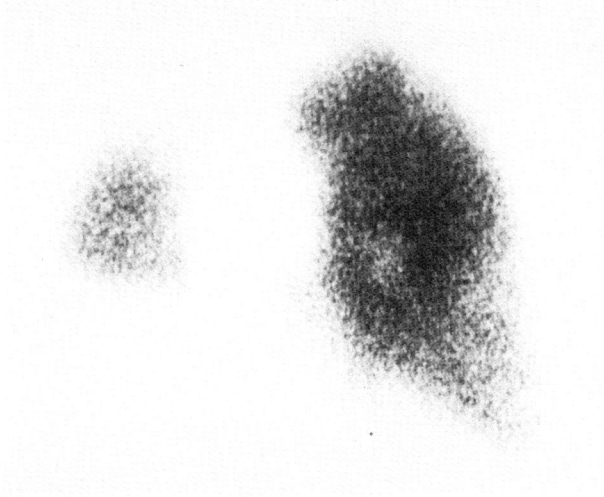

Figure 51*b*

Case 52

This patient was admitted with acute onset of severe dyspnoea. What is this investigation and what does it show? What other information should be obtained at the same time? What further investigations are required?

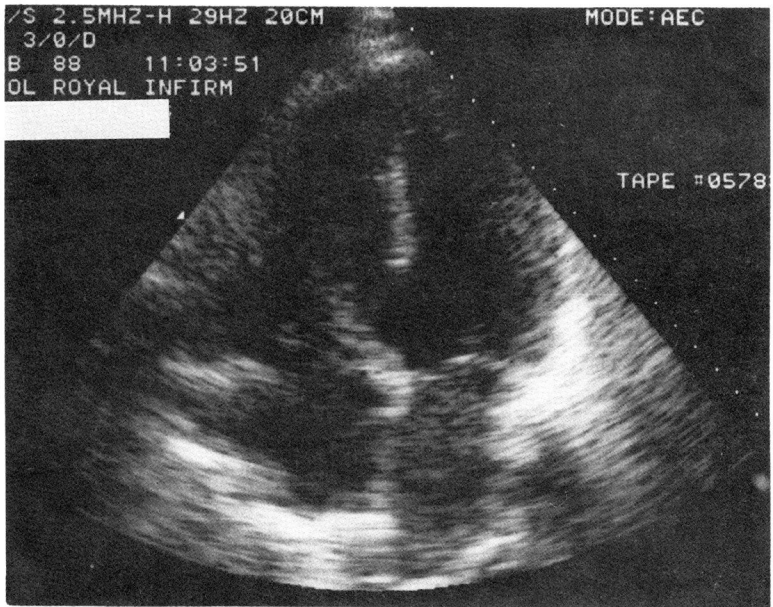

Figure 52

This is a 2-D Echocardiogram showing an optical four-chamber view of the heart, with the left ventricle on the right of the image. There is a large defect in the interventricular septum extending from just below the mitral valve ring into the muscular part of the septum. There is a flap of septum displaced into the right ventricle. This is the appearance of a Postmyocardial Infarct VSD. A Chest Radiograph was taken at the same time and showed evidence of severe pulmonary oedema and a left-to-right shunt.

These patients are usually very sick and as much information as possible should be obtained non-invasively by echocardiography. This should include assessment of Left Ventricular Function and Mitral Regurgitation (which may be present due to poor left ventricular function, chordal rupture or papillary muscle dysfunction). In some situations this is all the information that can be gained before the patient needs to undergo surgery. Coronary Angiography may be necessary to outline the extent of the coronary artery disease and to allow bypass grafting at the time of repair of the VSD. If the echocardiographic examination is complete left ventriculography and right heart catheterization is unnecessary and only prolongs a dangerous procedure. Giving contrast medium to these patients can make their clinical condition deteriorate rapidly and angiography should be limited to the minimum number of coronary artery injections required to show the extent of the coronary artery disease.

CARDIOVASCULAR SYSTEM

Case 53

These images were obtained in the left anterior oblique projection immediately after an injection during exercise (*Fig.* 53a) and in the same projection three hours later (*Fig.* 53b). What is the investigation and what does it show? What is the significance of this finding? What alternative forms of stress may be used as part of this investigation? What is the accuracy of this technique?

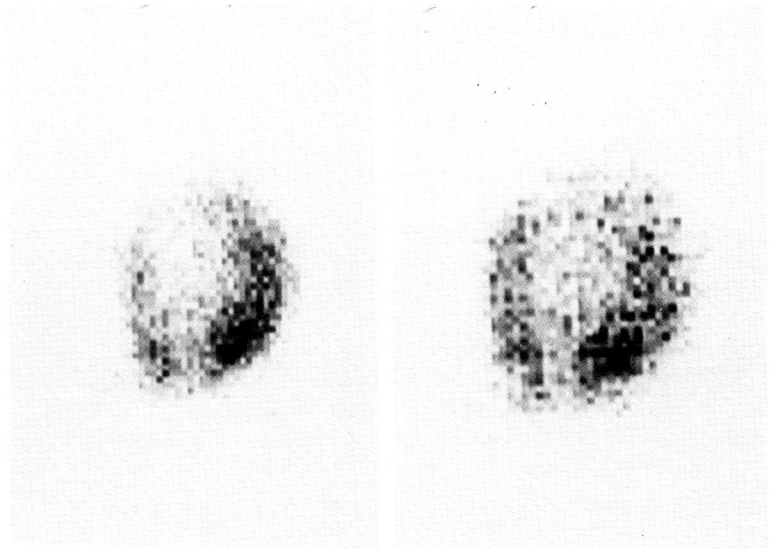

Figure 53a   *Figure* 53b

This is an Exercise Thallium Scintigram which shows a reversible perfusion defect in the interventricular septum. This indicates a significant Stenosis in the Left Anterior Descending Artery, which impairs perfusion during exercise. The usual form of stress used for this investigation is some form of exercise on a treadmill or bicycle. Alternative methods for producing stress include Vasodilators (i.e. Dipyridamole), Isometric Exercise and Cold Pressor Stress. These alternatives have a number of drawbacks, including a reduction in sensitivity of the test for detecting ischaemia.

The accuracy of thallium scintigraphy depends on a number of factors including the level of exercise achieved by the patient, the prevalence of ischaemic heart disease in the population under investigation and the extent of the disease (as interpretation of the images depends on having normal myocardium to compare with the abnormal area). Conventional exercise thallium scintigraphy has an overall sensitivity of 75–85 per cent and a reported specificity of 85–100 per cent, although the latter figure is probably not representative of the situation in most centres. When combined with single photon emission computed tomography (SPECT) and computer correction, compared with the normal population, reliable sensitivities in excess of 90–95 per cent can be achieved.

Thallium imaging is of particular value in assessing the functional significance of borderline lesions shown by angiography, in screening for coronary artery disease and in assessing the effect of treatment, such as angioplasty.

Case 54

What is this examination and what does it show? What are the therapeutic options? What are the potential hazards of these options?

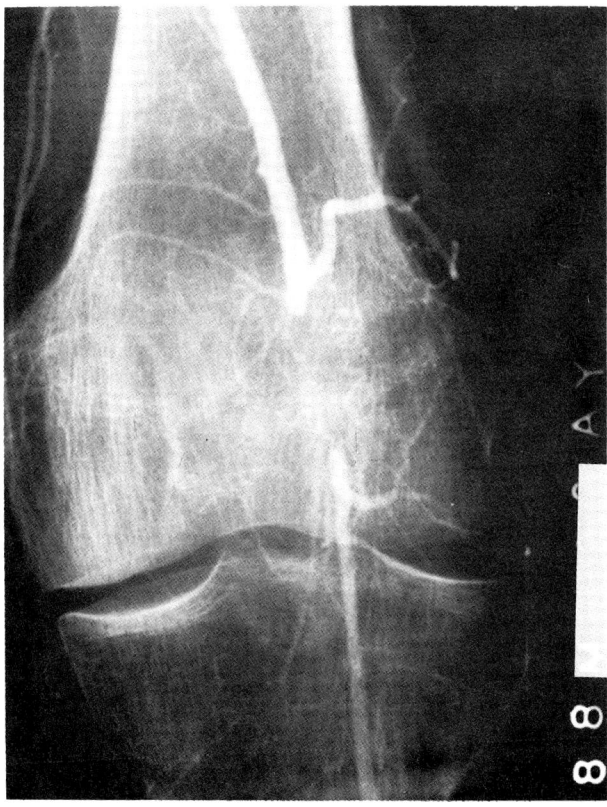

Figure 54a

This is part of a femoral arteriogram which shows a short Occlusion of the Popliteal Artery. The diagnosis of this can often be made non-invasively; angiography is performed as a prelude to treatment.

The majority of patients with short occlusions of this type have intermittent claudication and are usually treated, in the absence of severe disease elsewhere in the arteries of the leg, by the advice to give up smoking, lose weight and take more exercise. If symptoms justify more active treatment the alternatives include balloon angioplasty, laser recanalization, trans-catheter atherectomy and bypass surgery. The use of lasers and atherectomy devides is still in the experimental stage. Balloon angioplasty and bypass surgery generally have good results, the overall success of the procedure being related to the skill of the operator and the quality of the distal calf arteries. The hazards of angioplasty include damage to the femoral artery at the puncture site, dissection or rupture of the vessel at the site of dilatation, distal embolization and acute thrombosis. The hazards of surgery include those of anaesthesia in a group of patients with a high prevalence of carotid and coronary artery disease and graft occlusion due to anastomotic stenoses or poor flow due to poor distal run off.

This particular patient was referred for laser angioplasty after conventional angioplasty had failed. In spite of this it was felt that the lesion could be crossed with a guide wire only and this proved to be the case. The occlusion was successfully dilated (*Fig.* 54*b*) with a good clinical, haemodynamic and symptomatic result.

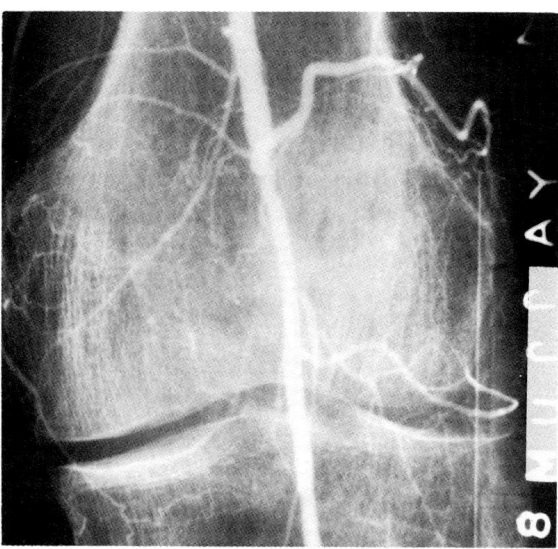

Figure 54*b*

Case 55

What abnormalities does this chest radiograph show? What is the likeliest diagnosis? What other investigations would you consider to confirm this diagnosis? The patient is 60 years old.

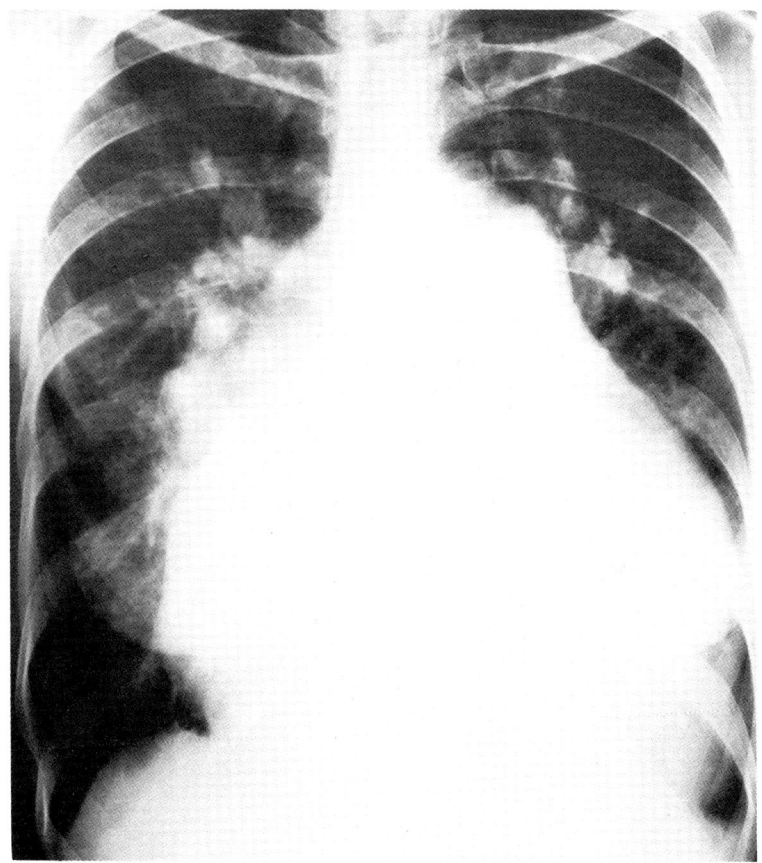

Figure 55

The heart is enlarged with a large main pulmonary artery and a small aortic knuckle. The proximal lobar pulmonary arteries are large but the peripheral pulmonary arteries are very small. The lungs are otherwise unremarkable. In a patient of this age the likeliest diagnosis is a Secundum Atrial Septal Defect. There is no evidence of left atrial enlargement which makes severe mitral valve disease unlikely (compare with Case 35). In a VSD the heart is unlikely to be this large (compare with Case 13).

The large heart, a small aortic knuckle and evidence of pulmonary hypertension are characteristic of this diagnosis and there are few reasonable alternative diagnoses except mixed mitral valve disease, when the left atrium should be visibly enlarged.

Echocardiography usually confirms the diagnosis but in this age group echocardiography may be difficult. Contrast echocardiography may be required in difficult cases when there is little flow across the ASD detectable with Doppler. Doppler can also give an assessment of pulmonary artery pressures and in skilled hands assess the degree of shunting. Alternative methods for confirming the diagnosis include first pass isotope scans, right heart catheterization with angiography (which will also give useful information on the degree of pulmonary hypertension) and magnetic resonance imaging, when available.

CARDIOVASCULAR SYSTEM

Case 56

This patient has intermittent pain in her left arm. What is this investigation and what does it show? Why is part of the image black and part white?

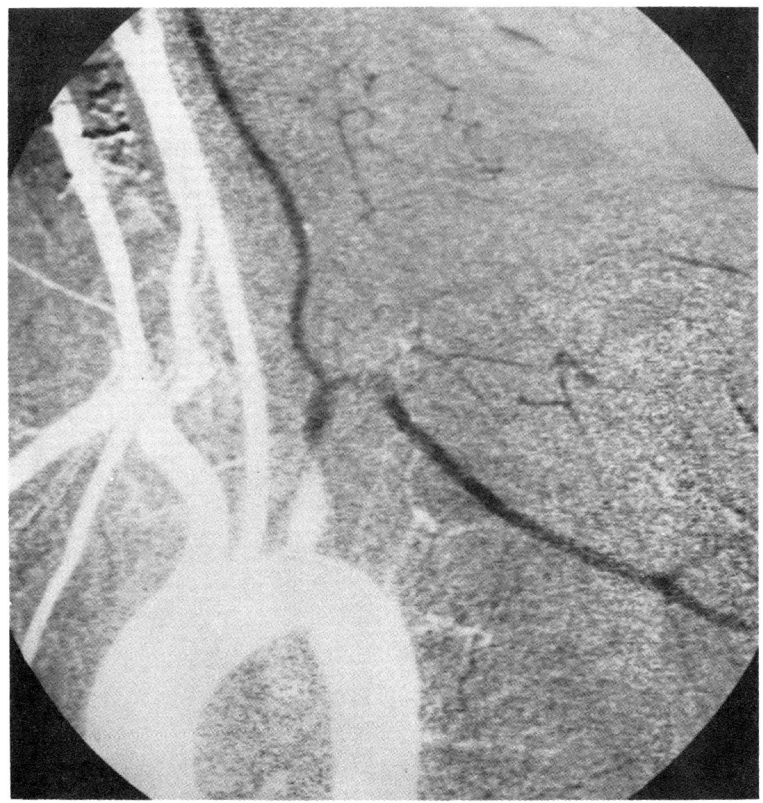

Figure 56

This is an Intra-arterial Digital Subtraction (i.a. DSA) Arch Aortogram which shows a severe short stenosis of the left subclavian artery. An early image with contrast in the arch of the aorta and carotid arteries has been used as a mask for the digital subtraction. A later image with contrast in the left vertebral and subclavian arteries has been subtracted from this. Because there is a difference in timing of the opacification of the vessels the early filling vessels appear white while the late filling vessels are shown as black. This image can be reversed electronically but the differences in phase or timing of filling, and therefore relative colour, remain.

The delay in filling of the left subclavian artery suggests that there is a 'Subclavian Steal Syndrome'. In this a severely stenosed or occluded subclavian artery derives its blood supply from retrograde flow in the vertebral artery, which enters the subclavian artery distal to the diseased segment. This may reduce the blood supply to the vertebral artery territory and cause symptoms of vertebrobasilar insufficiency. In patients with significant carotid artery disease the need to supply the arm by flow through the carotid and then vertebral arteries may lead to even more extensive cerebral hypoxia.

Case 57

This is the chest radiograph of a patient who is being followed up in the cardiology clinic. What abnormalities does it show and what is the most likely diagnosis?

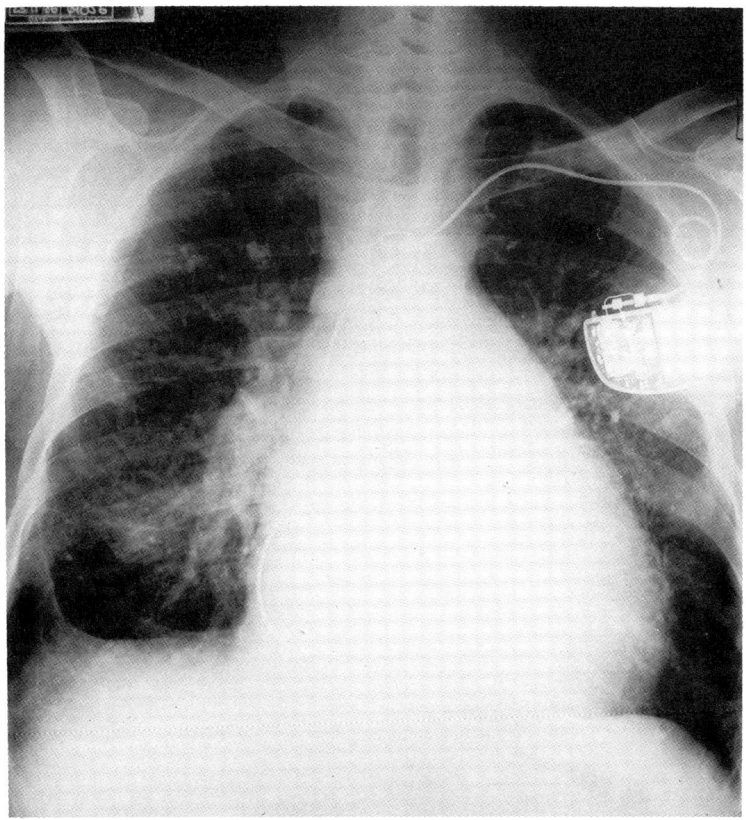

Figure 57a

There is a permanent endocardial pacemaker with a unipolar pacing wire, the tip of the wire is projected at the level of the right ventricular apex. The heart is enlarged and there is enlargement of the left atrium and the proximal pulmonary arteries. The peripheral pulmonary arteries are small and there are multiple calcific density opacities in both lung fields. At least one sternal suture wire is visible. These appearances suggest that the patient has had Chronic Mitral Valve disease with Pulmonary Hypertension and Pulmonary Ossification and which has now been treated surgically.

The sternal suture indicates that the patient has had cardiac surgery, most probably either a mitral valve replacement (confirmed by the lateral view, *Fig.* 57 *b*) or, less probably, an open mitral valvotomy. The presence of pulmonary ossification indicates that the pulmonary hypertension has been present for a long time. This type of chest radiograph should now be getting rarer as patients with mitral valve disease are diagnosed at an earlier stage. It is unfortunately still quite common to come across patients with radiographic evidence of mitral stenosis over a significant period of time in whom the diagnosis has been missed. Although there have been great improvements in the methods for detecting and assessing patients with valve disease the chest radiograph is still the most widely performed diagnostic imaging technique and provides important diagnostic information which is often missed.

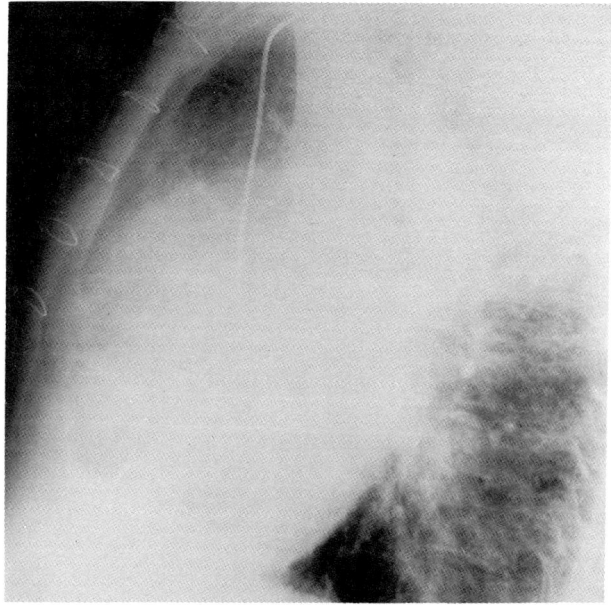

Figure 57 *b*

Case 58

This is the chest radiograph of a patient waiting for surgery for congenital cyanotic heart disease. What abnormalities are visible and what is the likeliest diagnosis? What are the alternative possible diagnoses? What further investigations are indicated?

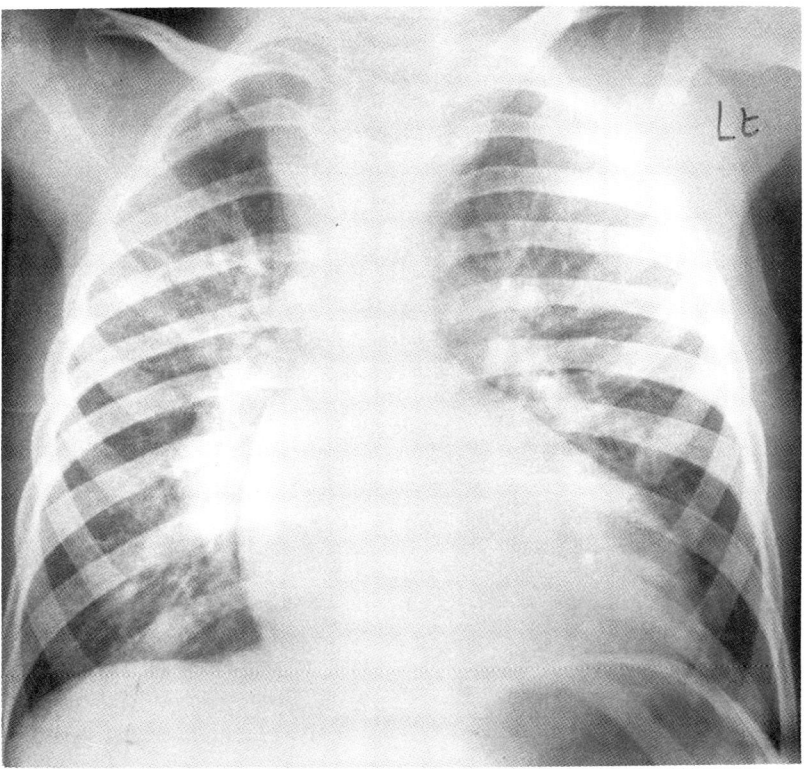

Figure 58

The heart is enlarged and there is a right-sided aortic arch. Although no main pulmonary artery is visible there is pulmonary plethora. There is no evidence of previous surgery. These features are strongly suggestive of Truncus Arteriosus, in this particular case the diagnosis was Type 1 Truncus.

Truncus Arteriosus is one of the more important causes of cyanosis associated with pulmonary plethora (others being uncorrected Transposition of the Great Arteries, Total Anomalous Pulmonary Venous Drainage, Single Ventricle). Forty to fifty per cent of patients with Truncus Arteriosus have a right-sided aortic arch, which is an uncommon association with any of the alternative diagnoses except single ventricle. In addition, the absence of a visible main pulmonary artery in its normal position may also suggest the diagnosis, although the main pulmonary artery is also obscured in patients with transposition of the great arteries. The right aortic arch, hollow pulmonary bay and elevated cardiac apex, commonly seen due to right ventricular hypertrophy, produce a classic appearance which is alleged to resemble a 'sitting duck'. The alternative diagnoses often have their own chest radiographic features which help with diagnosis, such as the 'Cottage Loaf' appearance associated with supracardiac TAPVD (see Case 48).

The diagnosis of Truncus Arteriosus is confirmed by echocardiography which will show a single truncal valve with a VSD and may show the origins of the pulmonary artery or arteries from the ascending aorta. Cardiac catheterization and angiography may be necessary to demonstrate the pulmonary artery anatomy and to measure pulmonary artery pressures before surgical repair. MRI can also make the diagnosis and may be sufficient to demonstrate the pulmonary arteries preoperatively in larger patients. The use of MRI is of course limited by its restricted availability.

Case 59

This is an image from an echocardiogram of an elderly patient who had presented with a stroke. What does it show and what is the likely cause? What alternative diagnoses should be considered?

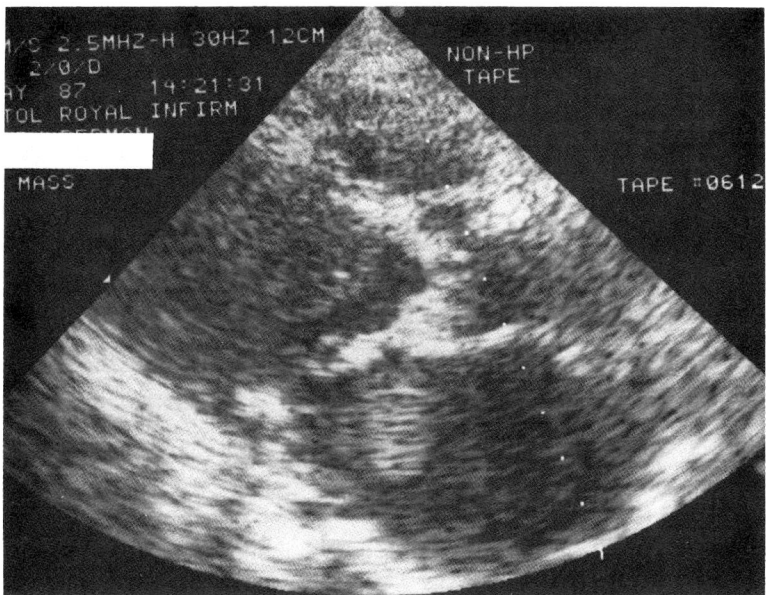

Figure 59a

The 2-D echocardiogram show that there is an echogenic mass in the left atrium and the left atrium is enlarged (over 4·5 cm diameter). In addition, the cusps of the mitral and aortic valve are thickened suggesting significant Aortic and Mitral Valve Stenoses. In the presence of mitral stenosis the mass in the left atrium is likely to be Thrombus and is the likely cause of this patient's stroke. The mass was very mobile (as indicated by the M-mode echocardiogram (→), *Fig.* 59*b*) and did not seem to be attached to the wall of the left atrium.

These very mobile thrombi are not only a potential source of emboli but can also obstruct the mitral valve orifice and cause syncope. The alternative diagnosis for this appearance would be left atrial myxoma but this tumour is rare and it is usually possible to see a point of attachment of the tumour to the wall of the left atrium, usually the lower part of the interatrial septum close to the region of the foramen ovale. Both these diagnoses place the patient at considerable immediate risk of suffering either severe systemic emboli, syncope or sudden death from occlusion of the mitral valve orifice. Such findings should be communicated urgently to allow surgical removal at the earliest opportunity.

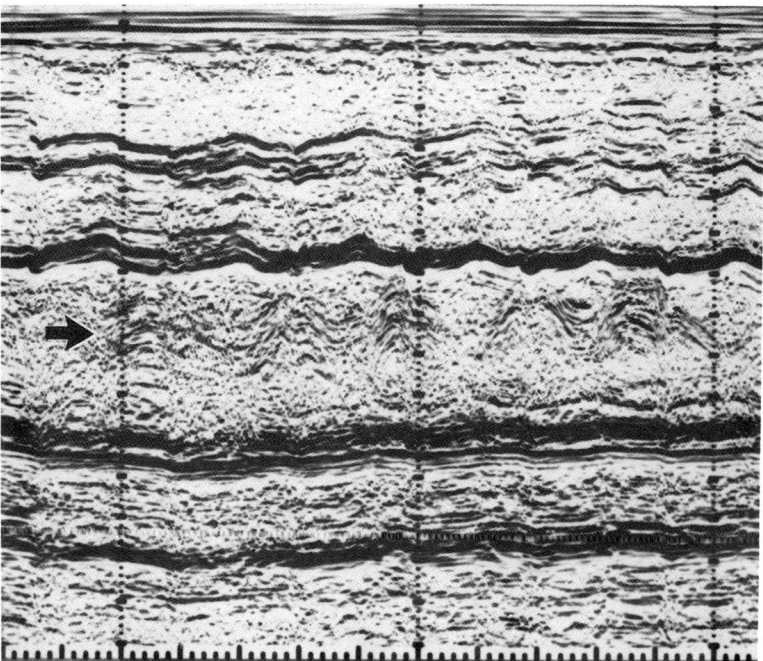

Figure 59*b*

Case 60

This patient recently had a diagnostic test as a hospital inpatient. Later the same day he complained of pain in the right leg. This investigation was performed. What is it and what does it show? How would you deal with this problem? What risk factors may contribute to the development of this problem?

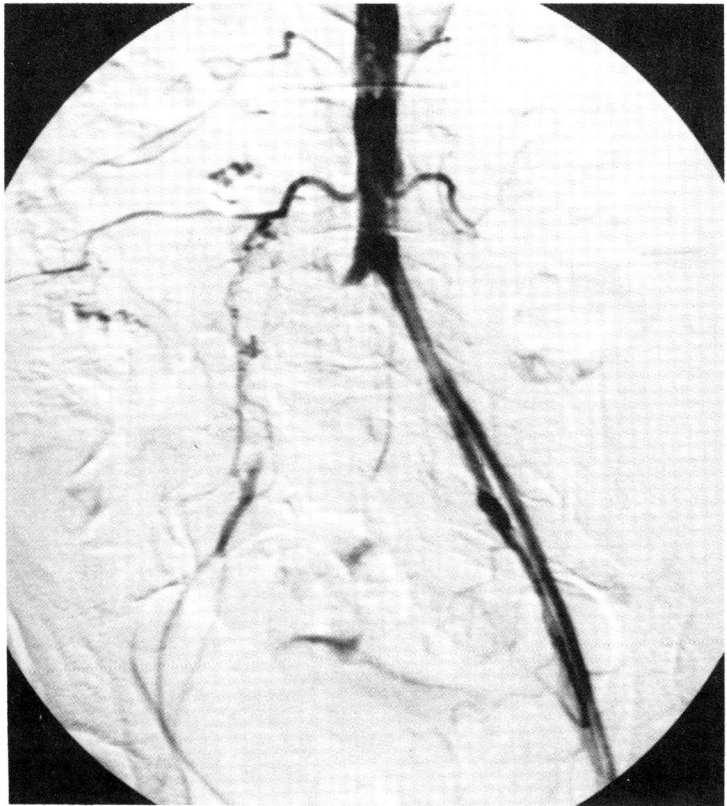

Figure 60*a*

This is an Intra-arterial DSA pelvic arteriogram, from the left femoral artery, which shows a Proximal Occlusion of the Right Common Iliac Artery. A short segment of the right external iliac artery is visible but apart from this there is little collateral vessel opacification. This indicates that the occlusion is recent and is probably related to the investigation carried out earlier in the day, an arteriogram from the right femoral artery, in this case a coronary arteriogram. This is one of the many complications which can occur following arteriography and emphasizes the importance of proper discussion of the risks of these procedures with the patient before the procedure. There are many other risks associated with arteriography which are related to the administration of contrast media, local vascular damage at the site of arterial puncture and damage to the organ under investigation. Local vascular complications include dissection, occlusion by thrombus and AV Fistula formation (as shown by i.v. DSA in *Fig.* 60*b*, which shows a post-arteriogram fistula between the left femoral artery and left femoral vein).

The treatment of this complication depends to some extent on the patient's condition and the circumstances under which the occlusion happened. A straightforward thrombotic occlusion can be treated with intra-arterial streptokinase, although if a more rapid result is required thrombectomy with a Fogarty catheter may be preferable.

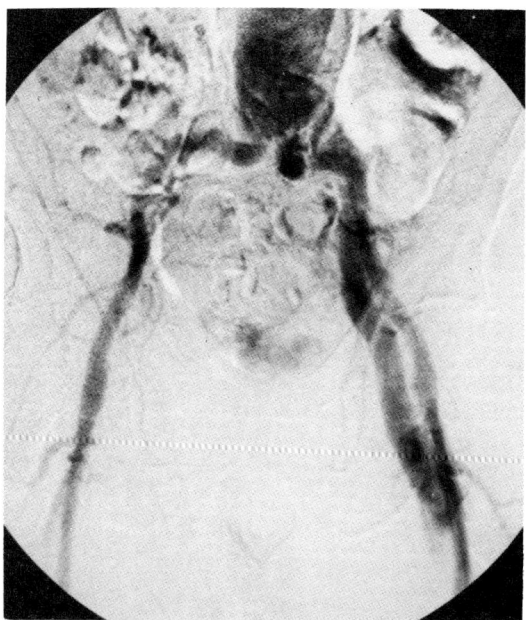

Figure 60*b*

Case 61

This is a contrast-enhanced CT scan of the abdomen in a patient who had a splenectomy one year before. What does it show? What are the possible aetiological factors which might produce this radiological appearance? What alternative imaging methods are suitable for making this diagnosis?

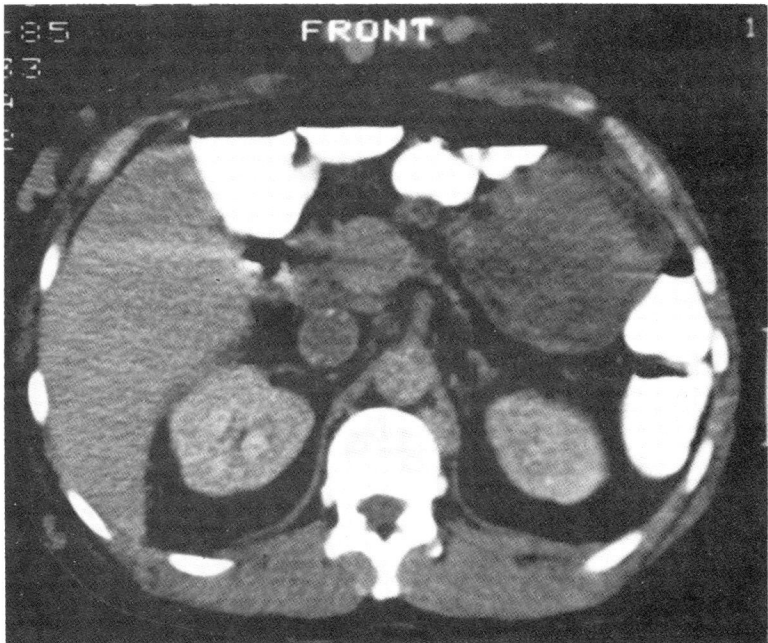

Figure 61

There is a mixed attenuation mass anterior and closely adjacent to the IVC. There is a mass between the spine and the left crus of the diaphragm which has the same attenuation as the aorta. This suggests that it is vascular. The IVC has a lower attenuation than the aorta indicating that it is thrombosed. There are a number of superficial masses in the patient's abdominal wall. These findings indicate Chronic IVC Thrombosis with the development of multiple dilated abdominal wall and retrocrural collateral vessels. The IVC thrombosis in this case may be related to the adjacent mass, the identity of which is not clear. In this particular Australian patient with hydatid disease there were a number of cysts more cranially, the mass shown here was an inflammatory mass which developed after splenectomy.

Other important causes of IVC thrombosis include:
1. Local inflammation (i.e. abscesses, lymphadenitis).
2. Local tumour (compression or direct invasion).
3. Trauma (including venous catheterization).
4. Extension of thrombus from peripheral venous thrombosis.
5. Surgical plication of the IVC or caval filters.
6. Hyperviscosity syndromes (i.e. polycythaemia, myeloma, thrombocytosis).
7. Pregnancy.

The alternative imaging methods include ultrasound with Doppler (ultrasound alone may commonly miss low echogenicity thrombus in the IVC), Isotope Venography (although this may have insufficient resolution to separate collateral vessels and the aorta from the line of the IVC), Ascending Venography (which carries a risk of dislodging thrombus) and MRI.

Case 62

What is this examination and what does it show? What confirmatory investigations are available and what are their complications?

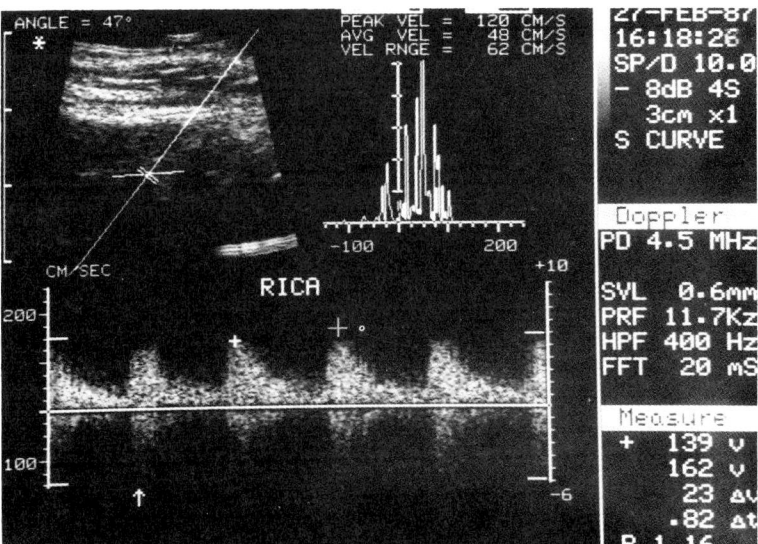

Figure 62a

This is a Duplex Doppler Ultrasound scan of the Right Internal Carotid Artery. It shows an abnormal flow pattern with an increased Doppler shift frequency indicating accelerated flow with spectral broadening and reversed flow elements (below baseline) indicating turbulent flow through a severe stenosis. Using any of a number of different diagnostic criteria this tracing indicates a stenosis of > 50 per cent reduction in luminal diameter.

The accuracy of Duplex Doppler in the assessment of carotid artery stenosis is often good enough to exclude severe stenosis (see also the discussion of Case 27). In patients with evidence of a severe stenosis where surgery may be an option, confirmation by some form of angiography is usually required, although there are some situations where some surgeons will operate on the basis of the Doppler examination only. Angiography should be performed by the safest possible method which will give adequate images (see Case 27). In the majority of patients good quality i.v. DSA, if available, will be satisfactory (as shown in *Fig.* 62*b*—the i.v. DSA carotid arteriogram in this patient showing bilateral internal and right external carotid artery stenoses).

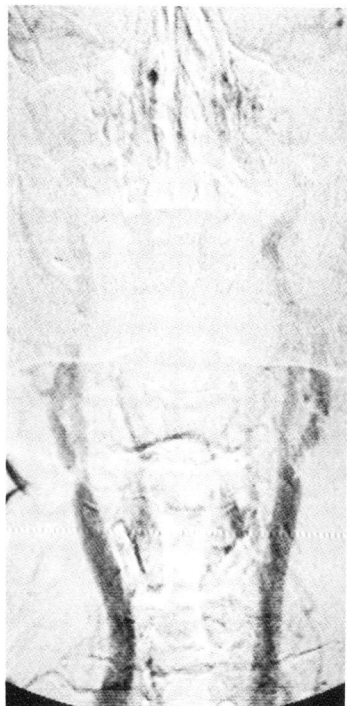

Figure 62*b*

Case 63

This 4-month-old boy was admitted for investigation of failure to thrive with poor feeding and tachypnoea. What does his chest radiograph show? What would your next investigation be? What is the differential diagnosis of this appearance?

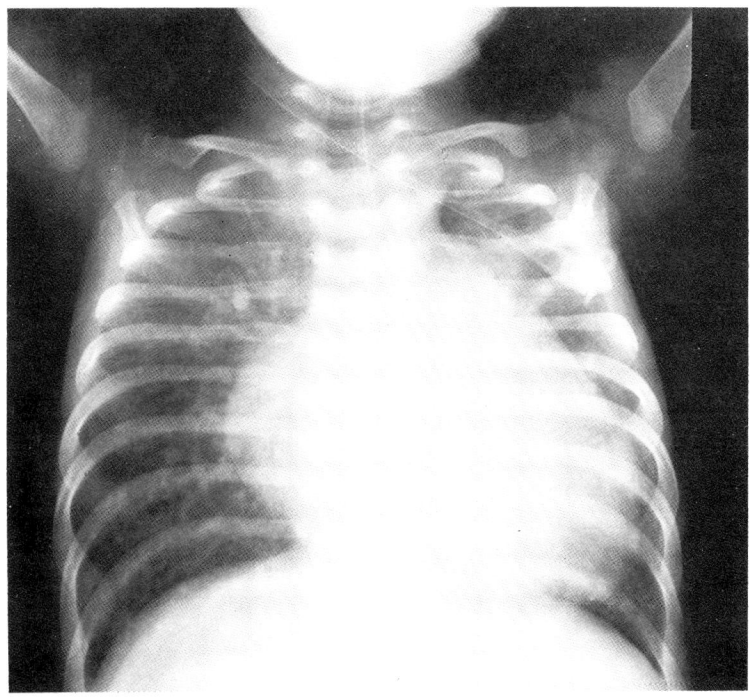

Figure 63

The chest radiograph shows a large heart with a left aortic arch, large main pulmonary artery and plethoric lung fields, indicating a significant (greater than 2 : 1) left-to-right shunt. There is, however, no evidence of pulmonary oedema. The next useful investigation, as in nearly all cases of children with congenital heart disease, should be echocardiography.

The differential diagnosis depends on whether the patient is cyanosed and you should have drawn up two separate lists of differentials, depending on the answer to this question. The differential diagnosis of pulmonary plethora in children with cyanotic congenital heart disease is discussed in Cases 48 and 58. This patient was not cyanosed and therefore the differential diagnosis includes:
1. Secundum ASD.
2. Partial anomalous pulmonary venous drainage.
3. VSD (which was the diagnosis in this patient).
4. PDA (see Case 33).
5. AV Canal defects. AV Canal defects are associated with mitral valve abnormalities (usually a cleft anterior leaflet) which lead to a degree of mitral regurgitation and may cause pulmonary oedema in addition to plethora.
6. Aortopulmonary window.
7. Gerbode defect (uncommon).

In children of this age it is not possible to distinguish reliably between these diagnoses on the basis of the chest radiograph appearances. The value of the chest radiograph is to demonstrate the presence of a left-to-right shunt.

Case 64

This 67-year-old patient presented with severe haemoptysis which required ventilation and blood transfusion prior to this investigation. What is this investigation and what does it show? What are the possible therapeutic options?

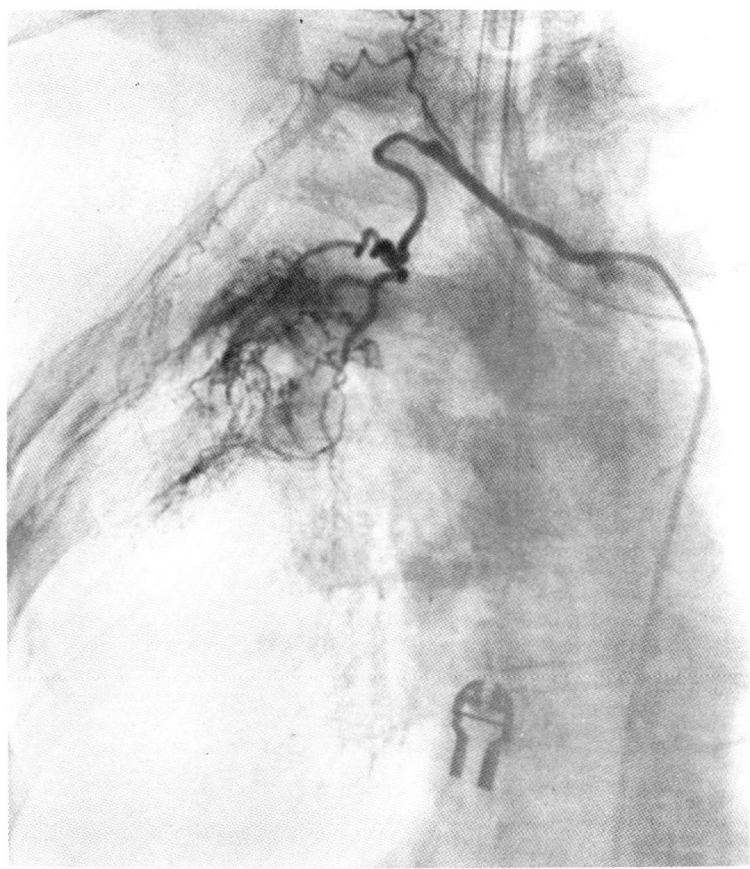

Figure 64a

This is a Selective Bronchial Arteriogram which shows multiple abnormal vessels in the right upper zone. In the midst of these vessels is an area of density which represents extravasated contrast medium which indicates active Bleeding from the Bronchial Artery. The original arteriogram (shown in *Fig.* 64*b*) has been enhanced by photographic subtraction, which subtracts the non-vascular structures, but there is enough detail to see that there is a double-lumen endotracheal tube which is selectively ventilating the left lung. This was protecting the left lung from being filled with blood from the right lung. There are abnormal right upper ribs and a chest wall deformity which indicate that the patient has had a right thoracoplasty. The bronchial bleeding is likely to be arising in an area of bronchiectasis or scarring left by the patient's previous tuberculosis for which he had a thoracoplasty.

This type of bleeding is difficult to control and requires either surgical or radiological treatment. In this case the patient had very poor respiratory function and was not fit for a thoracotomy. The bleeding artery was embolized with immediate control of the haemorrhage and rapid and sustained recovery. Severe bronchial artery bleeding of this type can also complicate bronchiectasis (particularly complicating cystic fibrosis), carcinoma, mycetoma, pulmonary abscess, idiopathic pulmonary haemorrhage and various other chronic fibrotic lung diseases and is often amenable to treatment by embolization.

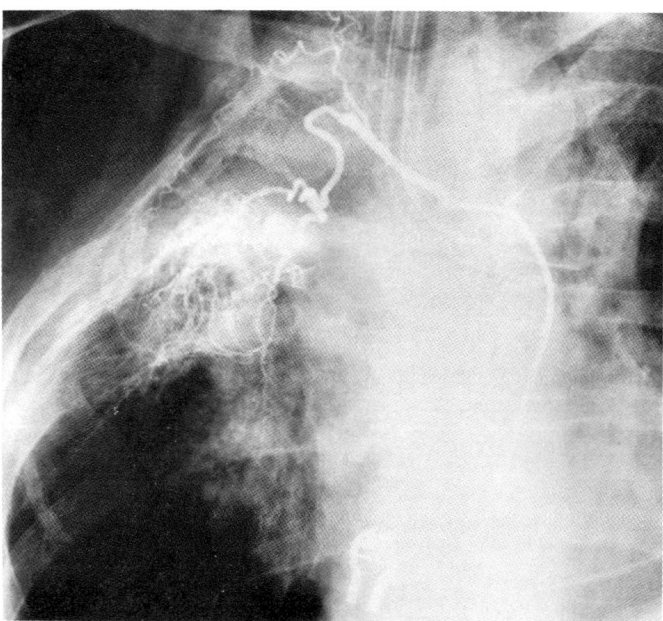

Figure 64*b*

CARDIOVASCULAR SYSTEM

Case 65

This is the chest radiograph of an elderly male patient who has been referred for assessment of his longstanding chronic obstructive airways disease. What abnormalities are shown on this radiograph and what is the differential diagnosis? What imaging methods are appropriate for establishing the diagnosis?

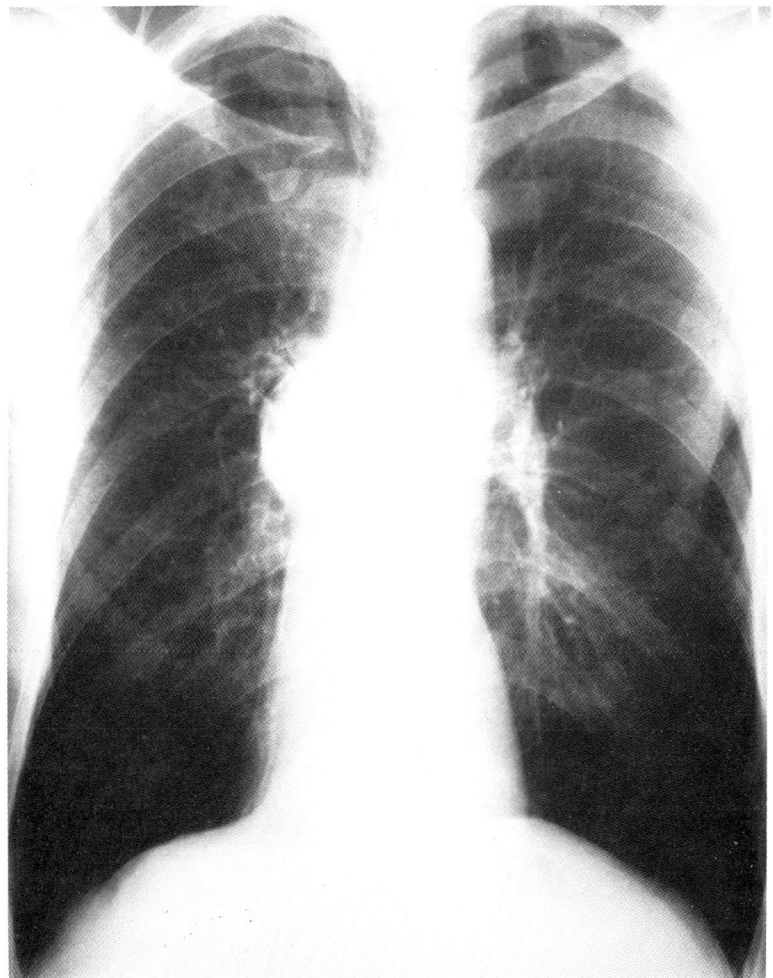

Figure 65

There is a smooth, rounded mass extending from the right hilum. There is a rim of calcification around the margin of the mass. The mass is in continuity with the right heart border indicating that it is situated in the middle mediastinum. The left hilum appears to be normal. The lung fields are of large volume with flattened depressed hemidiaphragms and a narrow mediastinum. The large volume lungs and the associated signs of hyperinflation are in keeping with the stated diagnosis of chronic obstructive airways disease. The unexpected abnormality shown on the radiograph is the right hilar mass. This has been localized to the right middle mediastinum and could be due to a number of differential diagnoses.

A mass in this region could be a Saccular Aneurysm of the Ascending Aorta, and this was the case in this patient. Round masses in this position with calcification in the wall can also arise in the pulmonary artery but are uncommon. The most common cause of a dilated calcified pulmonary artery would be longstanding pulmonary hypertension, as in an Eisenmenger Syndrome, but in such a case there should be bilateral changes. Rarely, Pulmonary Artery Aneurysms, as in Behçet's Disease, may calcify.

There are a number of causes of hilar lymph node calcification which could possibly mimic the appearance shown in this case. These include Silicosis (effectively excluded by the absence of any evidence of silicosis in the lung fields), Lymphoma treated by radiotherapy (although the calcification is often more generalized within the abnormal area) and rarely Sarcoidosis.

It is often said that calcification in an ascending aortic aneurysm indicates a possible luetic origin. This is true, and the appropriate investigations should be performed to exclude this diagnosis, but the likeliest cause of this appearance is now an atherosclerotic aneurysm. Saccular aneurysms of this type can cause complications as they expand by eroding through the chest wall or compressing other vascular structures in the mediastinum. Confirmation of the diagnosis is achieved by echocardiography, CT, DSA or MRI.

Case 66

This is an intravenous DSA arteriogram. What artery is under investigation and what does this image show? What further information is required from this investigation? What further investigation is advisable before treatment? What are the complications of this condition?

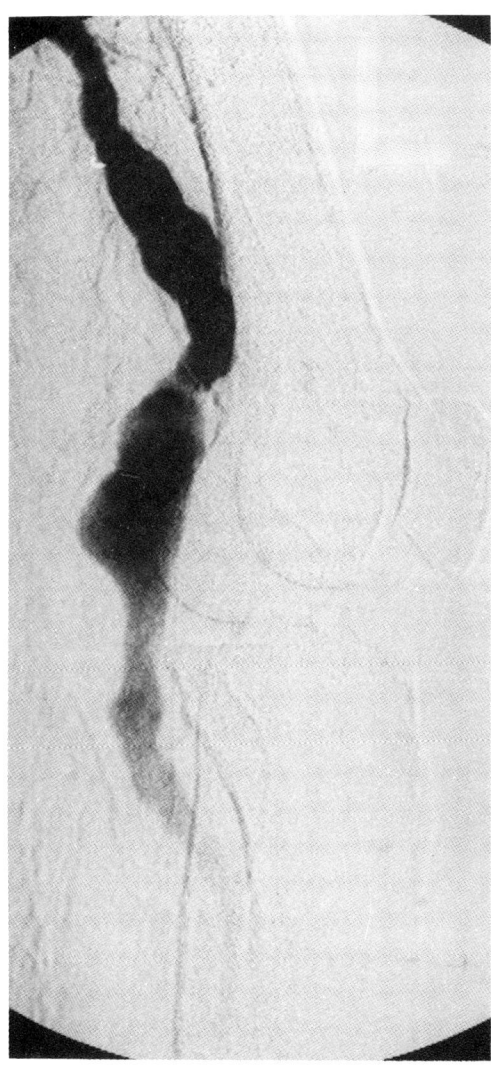

Figure 66

The arteries shown here are the Distal Superficial Femoral and Popliteal, shown in a lateral projection, as can be seen by the slight movement artefact which shows the knee joint anterior to the popliteal artery. There is tortuosity and dilatation of the distal superficial femoral and popliteal arteries. This is particularly marked at the level of the popliteal artery where it forms a Popliteal Artery Aneurysm. Further assessment by angiography should document the extent of the dilating disease so that surgery can deal with all of the abnormal vessel. It is necessary to demonstrate the level at which the distal arteries in the calf are normal and to confirm patency of these vessels before bypass grafting. This type of disease is often bilateral, as it was in this case, and the other leg also needs to be examined.

Popliteal artery aneurysms are often partly thrombosed and therefore the arteriogram may underestimate the size of the aneurysm. Ultrasound is an accurate method for assessing the overall size of the aneurysm and the extent of the thrombus within the aneurysm. In patients where surgery is deferred ultrasound is the method of choice for monitoring any change in size of the aneurysm which may indicate a need for surgical intervention.

The complications of popliteal aneurysms include:
1. Acute thrombosis with distal ischaemia.
2. Distal embolization.
3. Rupture.

CARDIOVASCULAR SYSTEM

Case 67

What abnormalities are shown on this radiograph and what is their aetiology? What are the treatment options which are now available for this condition?

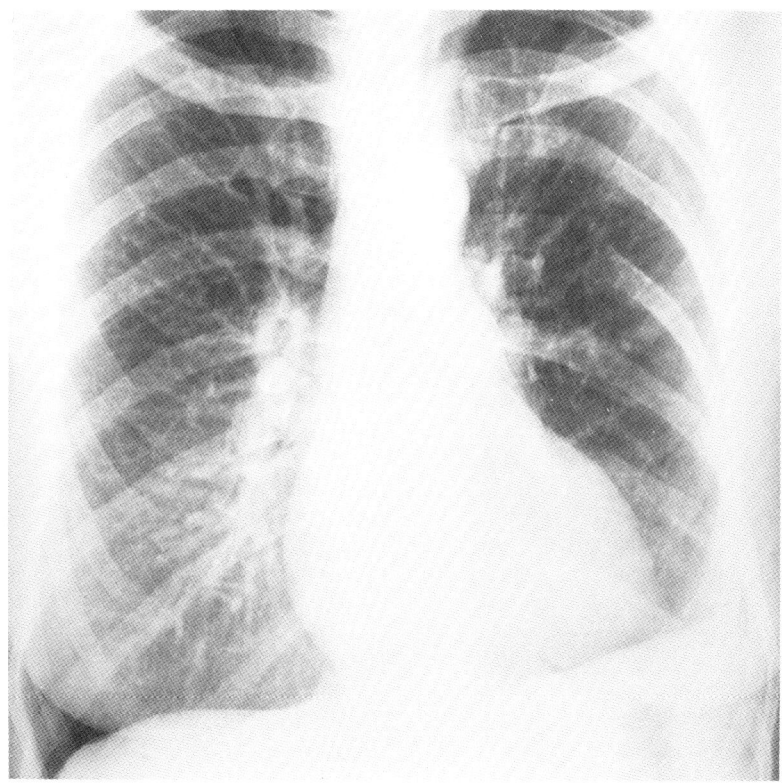

Figure 67

There is elevation of the left hemidiaphragm and pleural thickening at the left costo-phrenic angle. Part of the left seventh rib has been resected. The heart size is normal and has a normal shape with the exception of an area of indentation where the left atrial appendage should normally be visible. The lung fields are normal.

These appearances are characteristic of a patient who has had a Closed Mitral Valvotomy (which was performed via a left lateral thoracotomy). During this procedure the left atrium is opened through the left atrial appendage, which is subsequently closed at its base; thus there is often an indentation at that site on the postoperative radiograph. In patients who have had a closed mitral valvotomy (almost always for rheumatic mitral stenosis) look for evidence of prosthetic valves in both the aortic and mitral positions, which may be difficult to see in the density of the heart shadow on the frontal radiograph.

Closed mitral valvotomy is a very successful operation for mitral stenosis but does require open chest surgery. Techniques have recently been developed in which dilatation balloons, introduced using angiographic techniques, are used to dilate stenosed mitral, aortic or pulmonary valves (Percutaneous Balloon Valvoplasty—see discussion of Case 12). The initial results suggest that in patients with mitral stenosis the short-term results of this procedure are very good and the benefits of dilatation are sustained for at least several years. It seems likely that this technique will replace closed mitral valvotomy as the preferred treatment for mitral stenosis, particularly in those parts of the world where rheumatic heart disease is very common and there is limited access to cardiac surgery facilities.

CARDIOVASCULAR SYSTEM

Case 68

What is this investigation and what does it show? How was it performed? What are the possible causes of this condition?

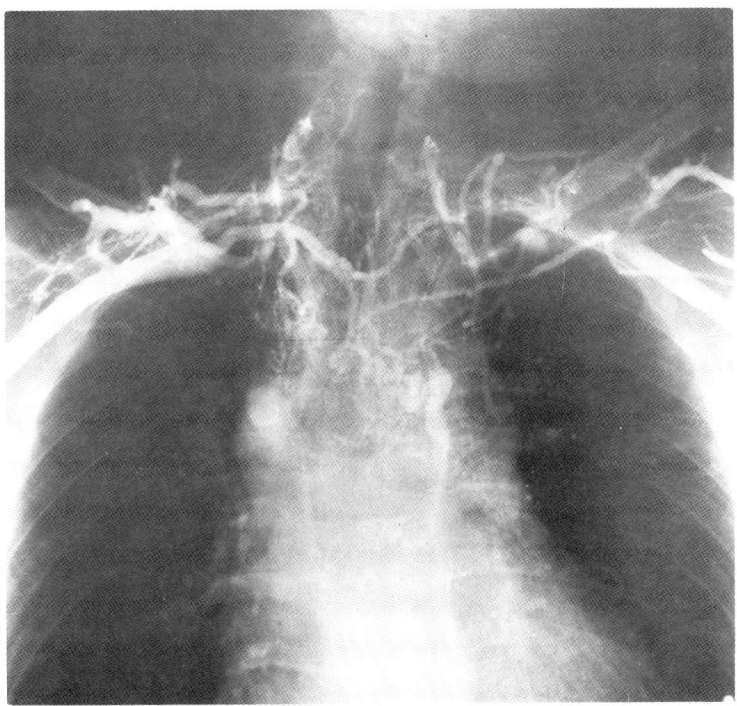

Figure 68a

This is a Superior Vena Cavogram which shows that there is no opacification of the superior vena cava. Contrast medium opacifies both distal subclavian veins, which drain into dilated collateral veins around the base of the neck and chest wall. There is opacification of the azygos and hemi-azygos veins. The diagnosis is Superior Vena Cava Occlusion, which is probably chronic in view of the well developed collateral veins shown on this image. This investigation is performed by inserting venous cannulae into veins in both arms, preferably a large antecubital vein, and injecting non-ionic contrast medium through both cannulae simultaneously. This allows demonstration of the proximal occlusions on both sides of the chest on the same film.

There are many causes of superior vena caval occlusion, the majority producing thrombosis. These include Mediastinal Malignancy, Radiotherapy, Mediastinal Sepsis, Fibrosing Mediastinitis (the cause in this case), peripheral or central administration of Irritant Infusion Fluids or Cytotoxic Drugs, and Central Venous Foreign Bodies (such as pacing wires, as shown in *Fig.* 68b, and central venous cannulae).

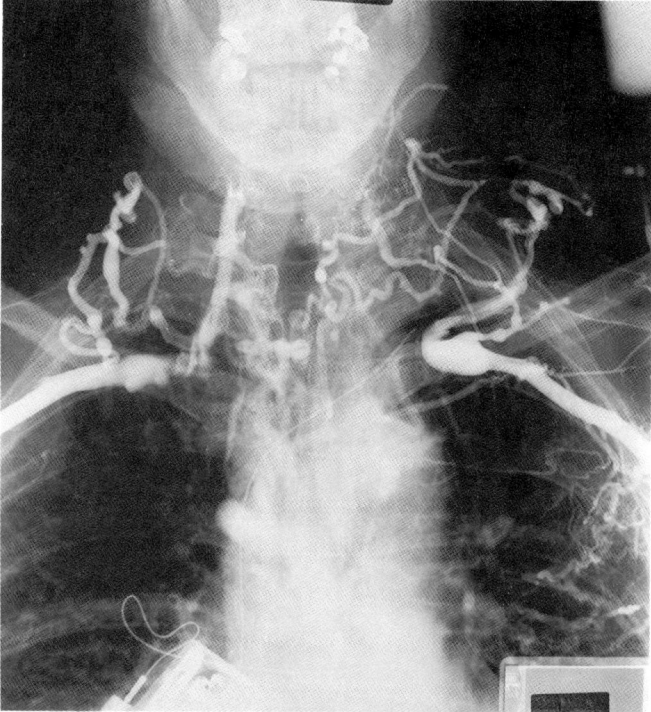

Fig. 68b

Case 69

This child presented within a day of birth with tachypnoea and increasingly severe cyanosis and acidosis. What does this chest radiograph show and what is the likely diagnosis? What treatment would have been used at the time of presentation?

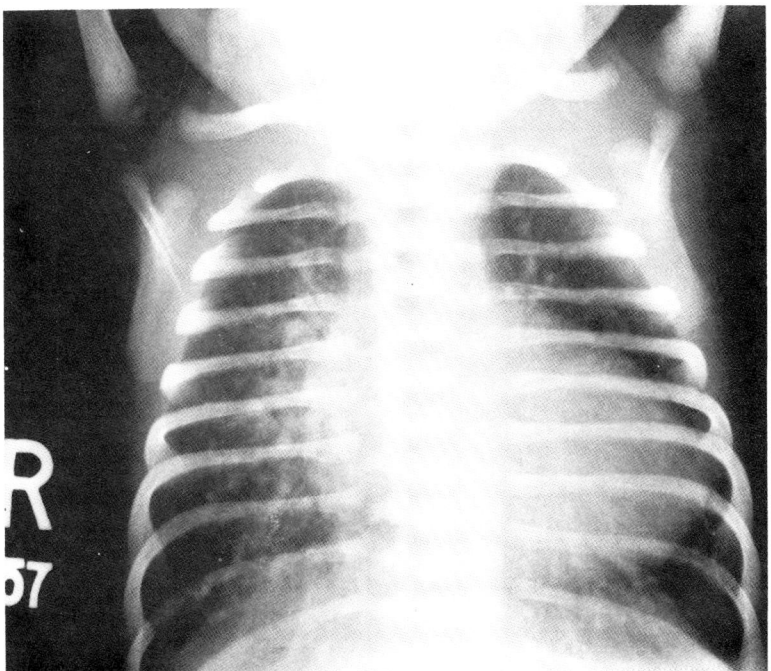

Figure 69a

There is a narrow superior mediastinum with a normal size heart, the apex of which is elevated, and a prominent right atrium. This resembles an 'egg on its side'. There is also pulmonary plethora. The differential diagnosis of cyanotic congenital heart disease associated with pulmonary plethora is discussed in Cases 48 and 58. The configuration of the heart is typical of Transposition of the Great Arteries.

The diagnosis is confirmed by echocardiography, and subsequently augmented by angiography (see *Fig.* 69 *b* which is a left ventriculogram showing the pulmonary artery arising from the left ventricle). These patients present at the time when the ductus arteriosus closes and initial management is to keep the ductus open using prostaglandins. Angiography is often performed at this time as it can be combined with palliative treatment (Rashkind Balloon Septostomy) which is aimed at re-establishing blood flow between the systemic and pulmonary circulations. Definitive treatment by Total Correction or an atrial diversion procedure (usually Senning operation) follows later.

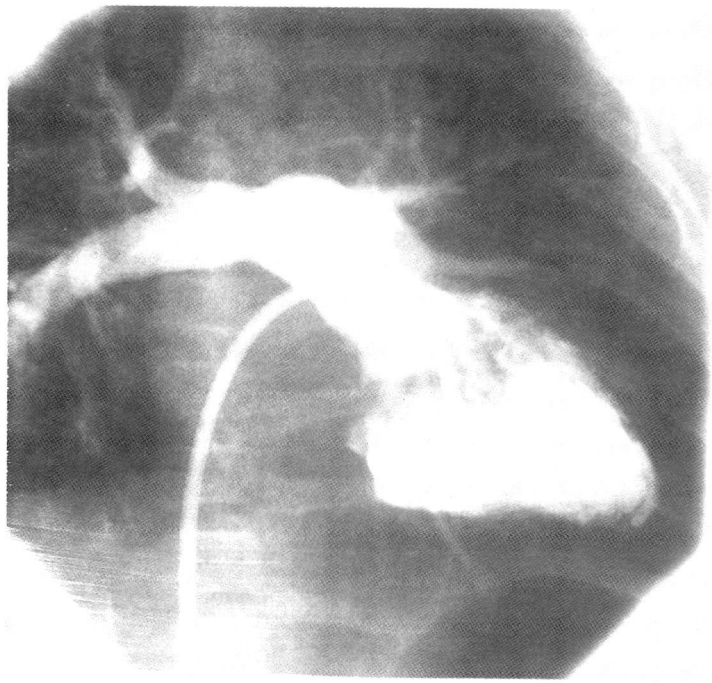

Fig. 69 *b*

CARDIOVASCULAR SYSTEM

Case 70

What does this examination show? What are the differential diagnoses? What other echocardiographic features may be present? What alternative methods are available to make the diagnosis and what do they show?

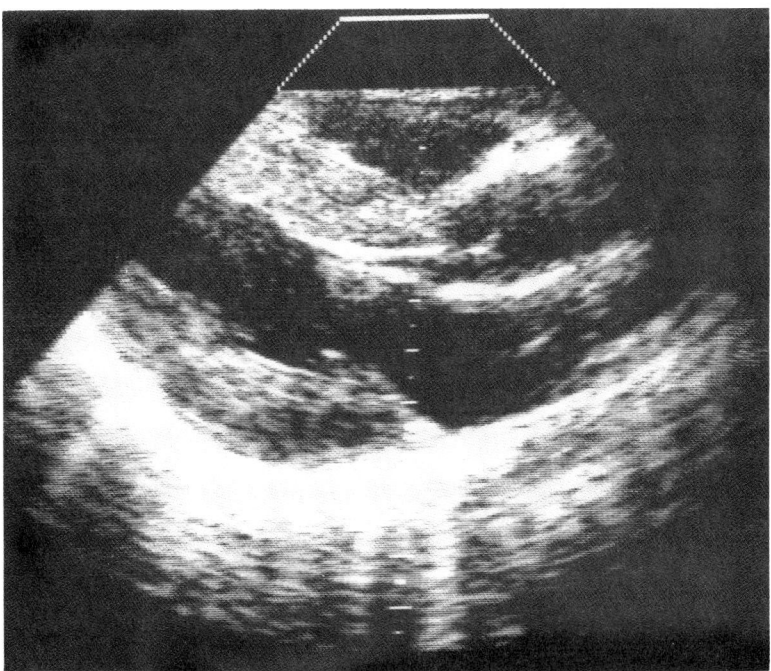

Figure 70

This is a diastolic parasternal long axis view from a 2-D echocardiogram which shows Hypertrophy of the Left Ventricle (both the posterior wall and the septum are approximately 2 cm thick). The mitral valve is open and the anterior mitral leaflet is touching the septum. The aortic valve closure line is clearly visible and the aortic valve appears normal. This makes one cause of left ventricular hypertrophy, Aortic Valve Stenosis, unlikely. The features of left ventricular hypertrophy are non-specific and are not diagnostic of any one condition. In the presence of a normal aortic valve this appearance could be due to Hypertension or to Hypertrophic Obstructive Cardiomyopathy (HOCM). In adult patients with aortic stenosis the aortic valve is thickened, has a reduced excursion and a gradient is detectable on Doppler at the level of the valve. In patients with HOCM a number of other signs are described but none of these alone is pathognomonic of the condition. These signs include midsystolic closure of the aortic valve, systolic anterior motion of the mitral leaflets (SAM) and asymmetric hypertrophy of the septum (ASH). These other features were also present in this normotensive patient who was therefore diagnosed as having HOCM.

Echocardiography is the most useful and readily available method for making the diagnosis of HOCM and excluding alternative diagnoses such as aortic stenosis. The diagnosis can also be made on the basis of an abnormal isotope ventriculogram (increased ejection fraction and small end-systolic cavity), CT (thickened ventricular walls), angiography (pressure gradient below the aortic valve and characteristic left ventricular morphology) and MRI (ventricular hypertrophy, small end-systolic volume, increased ejection fraction, systolic signal loss in the left ventricular outflow tract). Ventricular biopsy shows abnormal orientation of muscle fibres but even this is not totally reliable in making the diagnosis and is usually of research interest only.

Case 71

What is this investigation? For what conditions is it indicated? What does this particular case show?

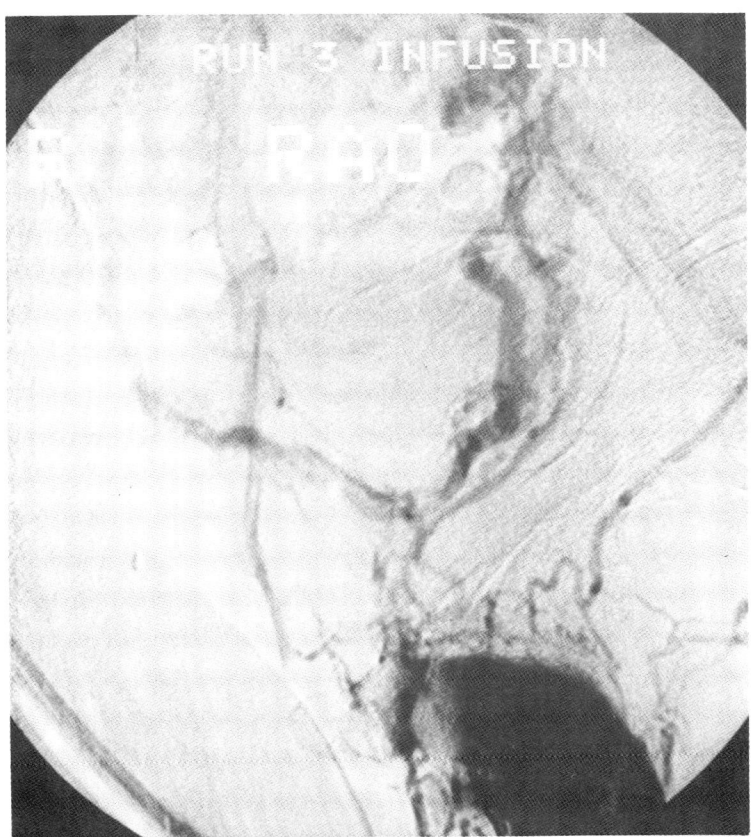

Figure 71a

This is a DSA Dynamic Cavernosogram, a procedure in which dilute contrast medium is infused directly into the corpora cavernosa to demonstrate the penile venous drainage and abnormalities of the corpora. This investigation is most commonly indicated in the investigation of organic Erectile Impotence but is also of use in the investigation of post-traumatic vascular problems and congenital or acquired penile deformities, such as those which occur in Peyronie's Disease.

This particular illustration shows marked opacification of the penile venous drainage, both deep and superficial veins, during an infusion of contrast. The veins are larger than on the control (pre-infusion) film (*Fig. 71 b*) and this indicates abnormal penile venous leakage. The penis is not erect. In a normal patient the veins seen on the control film get smaller or disappear during the infusion. Also in normal patients the penis becomes erect during the infusion.

Venous leakage is now widely accepted to be a common cause of erectile impotence. If arterial and psychosocial causes of impotence are excluded, by non-invasive testing and pharmacological provocation, venous leakage is probably the most likely cause of impotence. Cavernosography indicates the type of leakage and the appropriate type of surgical or radiological treatment.

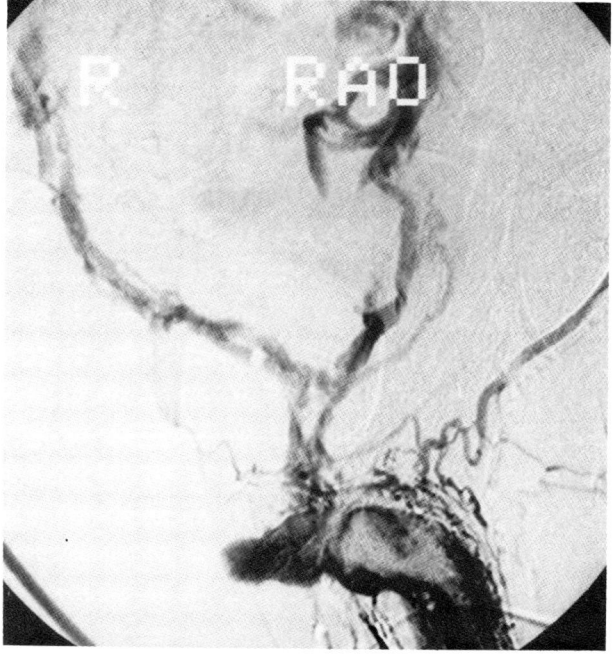

Figure 71 *b*

Case 72

This examination was deliberately performed to demonstrate simultaneously the trachea and the oesophagus. What does it show in this patient who was being investigated for stridor? What further investigations might be appropriate in this case?

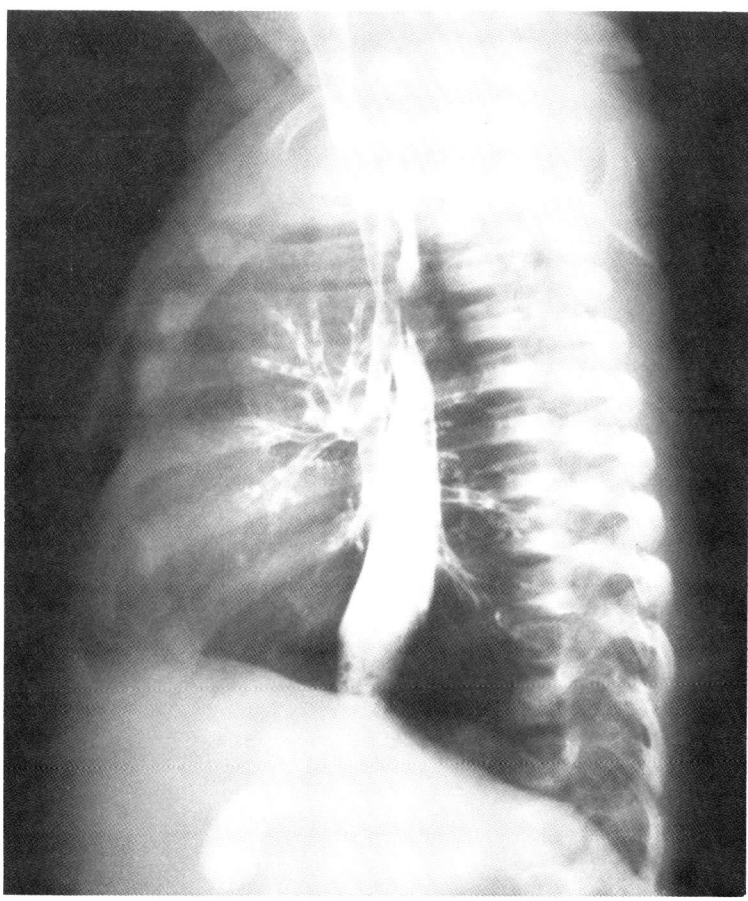

Figure 72a

This is a Bronchogram performed simultaneously with an Oesophagogram using an emulsion contrast medium. There is a posterior indentation on the oesophagus and the trachea just above the level of the carina. Simultaneous demonstration of both structures confirms that there is no abnormal structure (such as a vascular ring) between them and that the normality is situated posterior to the oesophagus. In this context the likeliest cause of this appearance is an aberrant right subclavian artery and this was confirmed by angiography (*Fig.* 72*b* is a subtraction angiogram showing the right subclavian artery arising distal to the origin of the left subclavian artery). Although other mediastinal masses can cause posterior indentation they are unlikely to cause such a short segment of narrowing at this level. A CT scan will show such masses but in small children CT can miss vascular rings and aberrant vessels, making angiography necessary to confirm or exclude their presence. The use of DSA can make the demonstration of these by an intravenous injection less invasive than conventional aortography.

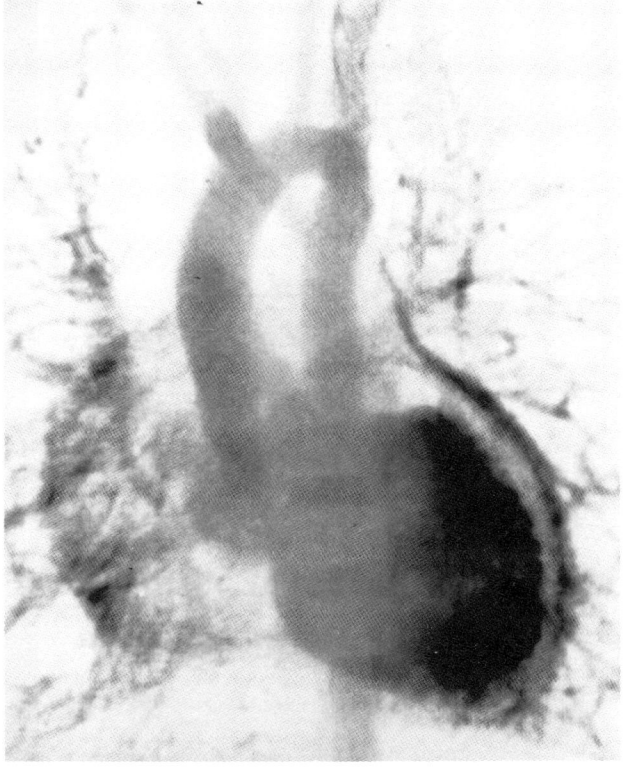

Figure 72*b*

CARDIOVASCULAR SYSTEM

Case 73

What is this investigation and what does it show? How should this lesion be treated? What other conditions are associated with this condition? What alternative imaging methods are suitable for establishing the diagnosis?

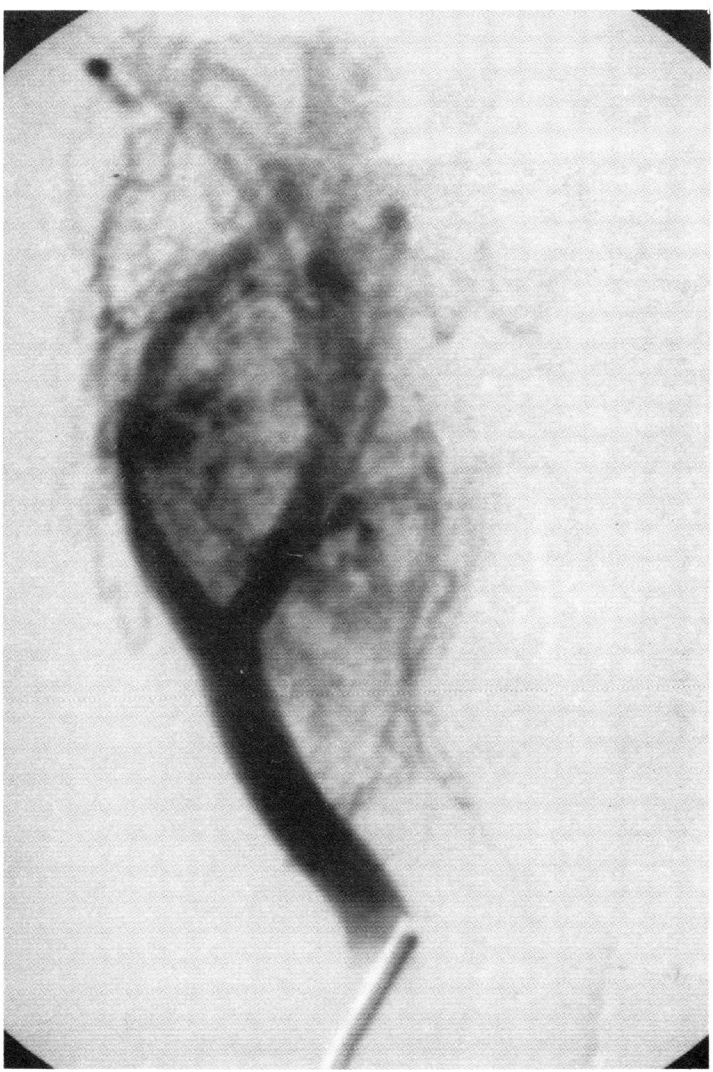

Figure 73 (By courtesy of Professor D. J. Allison)

This is a Selective DSA Carotid Arteriogram which shows an abnormal vascular blush around the carotid bifurcation. There is an abnormally wide angle to the carotid bifurcation indicating that the vascular mass is pushing the external and internal carotid arteries apart. Both of these vessels are patent. These are the features of a Carotid Body Tumour.

These tumours are not benign and can metastasize locally and, less often, distantly. The tumours grow slowly and become increasingly inseparable from the carotid arteries. They are seldom radiosensitive and for this reason surgical excision is the treatment of choice. The tumours tend to be very vascular and embolization shortly before operation can reduce their vascularity and make surgery significantly easier.

These tumours are usually unilateral. When they are bilateral there is a strong relationship with phaeochromocytomas, which may not be situated in the adrenals but elsewhere in the abdomen or mediastinum.

Alternative imaging methods for demonstrating Carotid Body Tumours include ultrasound (low echogenicity masses between the carotid arteries) and CT (enhancing masses at the carotid bifurcation causing separation of the carotid arteries). In some cases there may be further lesions around the base of the skull which ultrasound cannot visualize but which are well shown on CT and angiography.

Case 74

What is this investigation and what does it show? In what way is it incomplete? What further investigations are indicated?

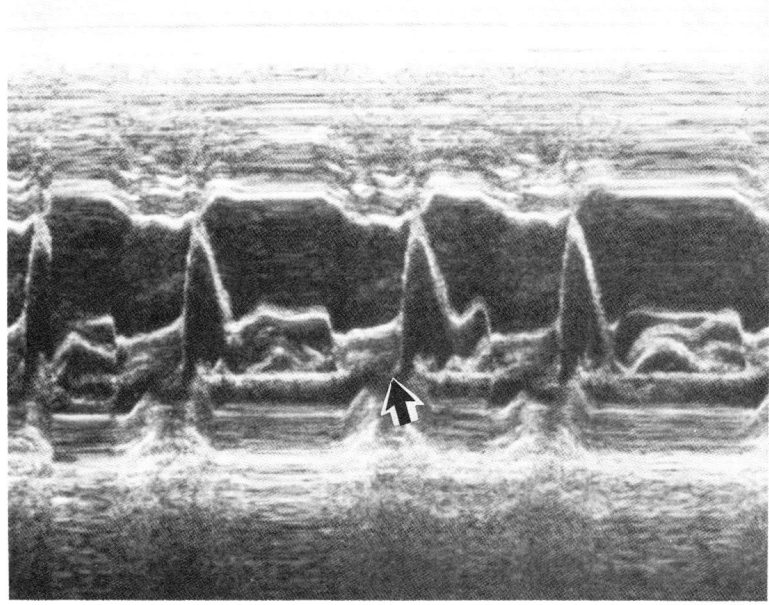

Figure 74a

This is an M-mode Echocardiogram which shows prolapse of the posterior mitral valve cusp (↑). The examination is incomplete as it does not include the patient's ECG, which is essential for accurately timing cardiac events on the tracing. The M-mode findings should be confirmed by 2-D. Echocardiography (*Fig.* 74*b* is the parasternal long axis image from this patient showing the prolapsing cusp at end-systole) and any associated mitral regurgitation documented with Pulsed Doppler. Left ventricular function should also be assessed by echocardiography.

Mitral valve prolapse is a common condition in otherwise normal patients but is not as common as was once suggested (up to 22 per cent of young healthy females in one series). It is thought that this abnormally high incidence resulted from difficulties in interpreting the M-mode signs of prolapse (posterior motion of one or both mitral cusps at some stage of systole, often associated with a variable degree of cusp thickening). The prevalence of prolapse is much lower when 2-D echocardiography is used and this should be used to confirm the diagnosis, rather than relying on the M-mode findings only. On 2-D echocardiography the prolapse of the cusps into the left atrium is visible (*Fig.* 74*b*) along with the thickening of the valve cusps due to myxomatous degeneration of the valve tissue. This is associated with an increased risk of systemic emboli.

Mitral valve prolapse is a common feature of Marfan's syndrome when it has a significantly worse prognosis than in otherwise normal individuals.

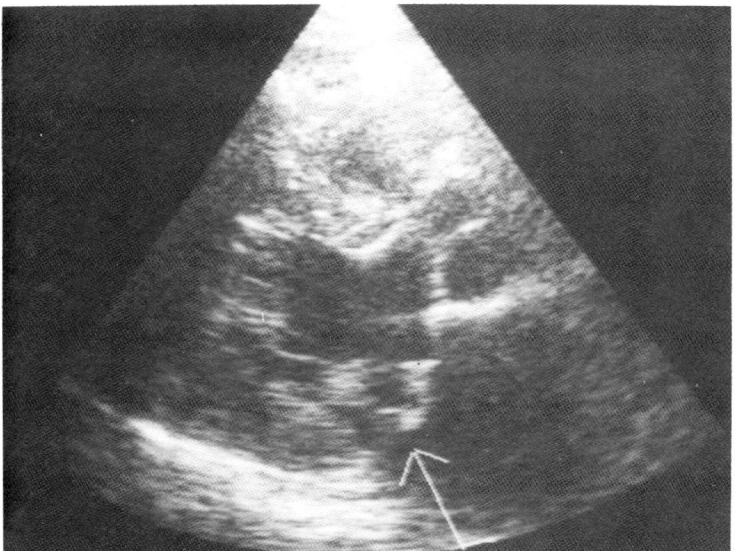

Figure 74*b*

Case 75

This examination was performed on a 41-year-old female patient who was admitted with a four-week history of dyspnoea and a five-day history of fever and increasing central chest pain. What is the investigation and what does it show?

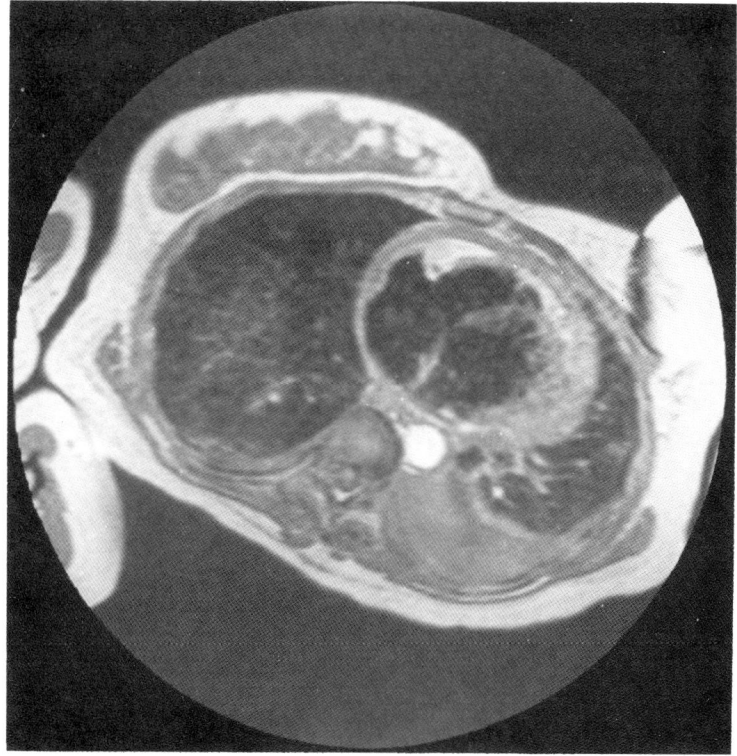

Figure 75

This is a Spin Echo Cardiac Gated MRI scan taking a transverse section through the heart. It shows an extensive pericardial effusion (mid-grey) surrounding the heart and a moderate left pleural effusion. Although pericardial effusions are usually very well shown by echocardiography this technique may have difficulty in showing the full extent of an effusion. This is especially so when the effusion is purulent and contains organizing fibrinous fluid, as in this case where pericardiocentesis confirmed the presence of a very viscous purulent pericardial effusion. A similar appearance could also be produced by pericardial thickening/ constriction and, if the thickening was more localized, pericardial tumours. Echocardiography also showed the presence of the pericardial effusion but its full extent was difficult to determine due to the high echogenicity of the purulent fluid, which appeared similar to myocardium in some areas.

Gated MRI scanning techniques are very useful in showing cardiac anatomy and can be orientated in almost any required plane. On this type of sequence fat and static blood (descending aorta in this image) have a high signal (white), muscle and viscous fluids (myocardium, organizing effusion) have medium signal intensity (grey), air and moving blood (in the heart in this very early systolic image) have no signal and appear black.

MRI is unlikely to replace echocardiography and angiography in the assessment of most cardiac disease in the immediate future. However, its ability to provide ECG gated scans in multiple planes with good contrast between blood and the surrounding tissues have already made it superior to CT scanning in the assessment of pericardial and aortic disease.

CARDIOVASCULAR SYSTEM

Case 76

This child has very recently had cardiac surgery. What does this chest radiograph show and what should be your next course of action?

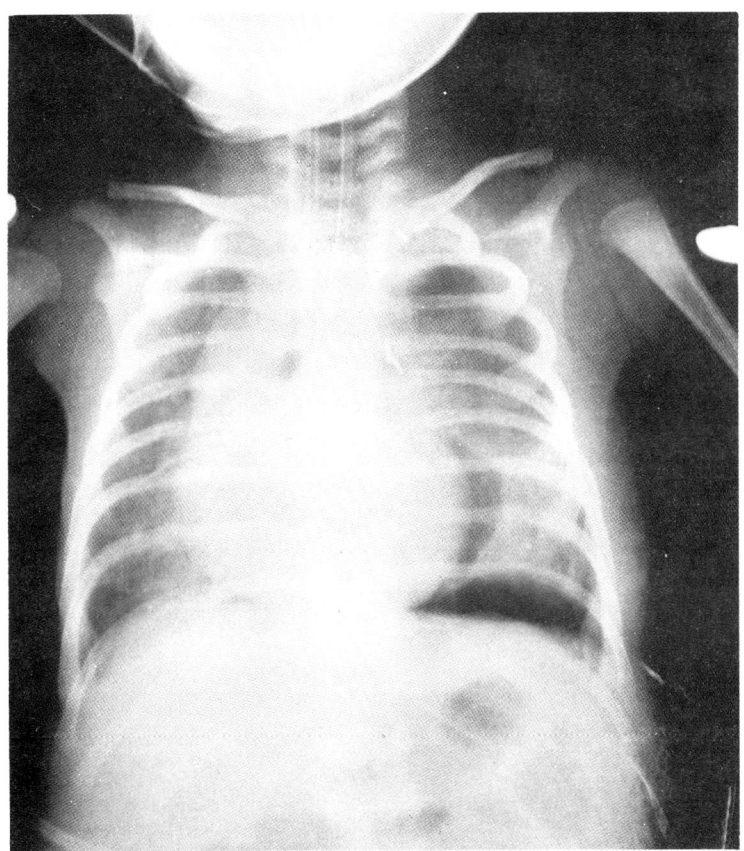

Figure 76a

There is air in the pericardium clearly outlining the heart, unlike mediastinal air which tracks along tissue planes and is less well circumscribed. In addition to the Pneumopericardium there is a left pneumothorax (seen most clearly above the left hemidiaphragm) and the endotracheal tube is deviated to the right. Although the patient's head is turned to the right the thorax is well centred and this cannot account for the mediastinal shift. This indicates that although the left lung is not completely collapsed there is a Tension Pneumothorax. There is also consolidation of the left lung, which prevents the lung from collapsing even in the presence of a tension pneumothorax. There is widening of the left third intercostal space indicating the site of the recent thoracotomy when the patient had a coarctation repaired (note the surgical clips adjacent to the left side of the mediastinum). Your next action is aimed at urgently relieving the tension pneumothorax. In this case this was not done until the appearance on the chest radiograph shown in *Fig.* 76*b* was seen, which shows considerable mediastinal shift to the right and further collapse of the left lung.

Pneumopericardium and tension pneumothorax are important conditions complicating ventilation in infants. In children with non-compliant lungs the radiographic features of tension may be masked. The presence of a pneumopericardium indicates that there is a significant air leak and this should stimulate an urgent search for evidence of a tension pneumothorax. In a ventilated patient in whom the pericardium has not been opened the presence of a pneumopericardium is associated with a high mortality.

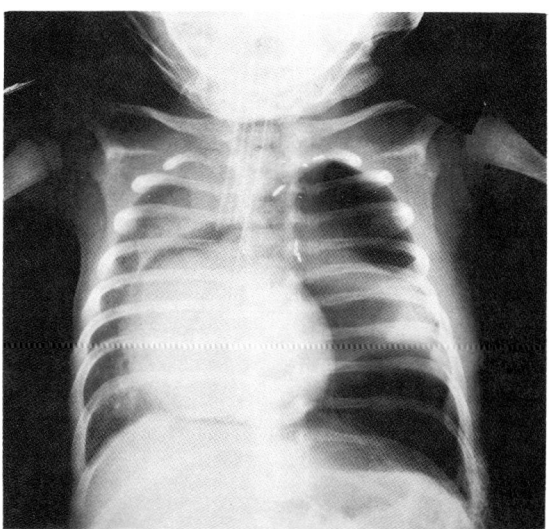

Figure 76*b*

Case 77

This patient was admitted for abdominal surgery and this chest radiograph was taken. What abnormality is shown and what is the differential diagnosis? What further investigations would you advise to determine the nature of the abnormality?

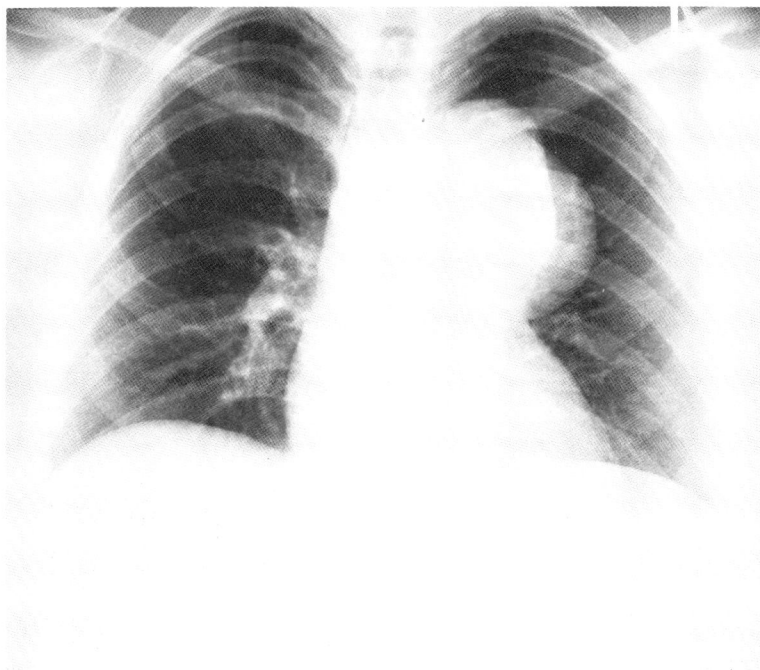

Figure 77

There is a lobulated mass extending from the left hilum which is well defined laterally but poorly defined medially. The wall of the mass is not obviously calcified. The lack of a border between the mass and the mediastinal structures such as the aortic arch and pulmonary artery localizes the origin of this mass to the middle mediastinum. The heart is not enlarged and the lung fields are normal. The likely differential diagnoses depend to a certain extent on the patient's history. An appearance like this could be seen with an Aortic Aneurysm which could be due to Atheromatous Disease, Syphilis or could occur following bypass grafting (often a Mycotic Aneurysm) and other chest trauma. The appearance could be due to Hilar Lymphadenopathy (particularly due to secondary malignant disease or lymphoma), Primary Mediastinal Tumours (benign such as teratomas, thymomas, fibromas, lipomas and their malignant equivalents).

The most useful examination to make a definitive diagnosis in this situation is usually a Contrast Enhanced CT Scan (or if available MRI). In this case the mass was initially thought to be an aortic aneurysm but at surgery was found to be a bronchogenic cyst. This case shows the importance of not prematurely reaching a conclusion about the pathological nature of a lesion when the radiographic findings only give non-specific information on the site and size of the abnormality. In the absence of any other information (clinical or radiological) it is then only possible to give a differential diagnosis with an indication of the likely probability of the various alternatives.

CARDIOVASCULAR SYSTEM

Case 78

This young child presented with symptoms of increasing heart failure with tachypnoea and poor feeding but no cyanosis. What does this chest radiograph show and what is the differential diagnosis? Are there any features you would look for on a chest radiograph which might favour one of these diagnosis?

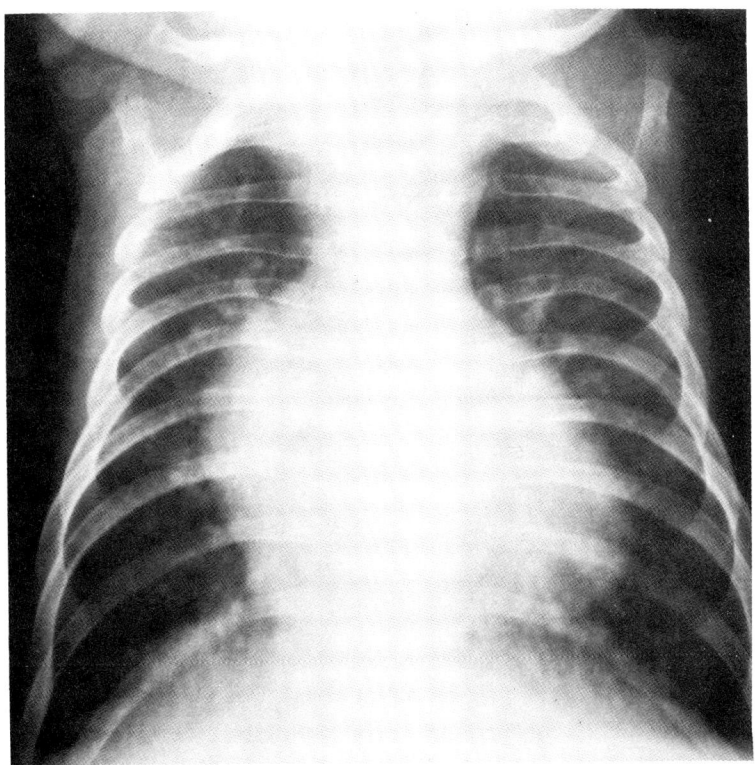

Figure 78*a*

This chest radiograph shows mild enlargement of the heart with a prominent right heart border suggesting that there is right atrial enlargement. The cardiac apex is elevated and the appearances would be consistent with a diagnosis of transposition of the great arteries. However, the child presented with heart failure but no cyanosis, making transposition relatively unlikely. The lung fields are plethoric and this indicates a significant left-to-right shunt. Although a VSD and PDA could be the cause they would not explain the enlarged right atrium, which indicates increased flow at atrial level. Uncomplicated ASDs seldom present at this age and seldom with heart failure. The large right atrium and the presentation in heart failure suggest a more complex shunt at atrial level with possible mitral valve deformity, in other words a form of Endocardial Cushion Defect (Ostium Primum ASD or Persistent Atrioventricular Canal Defect). Endocardial cushion defects are associated with a varying degree of mitral valve malformation, usually a cleft in the anterior mitral leaflet (as shown in the 2-D echocardiogram illustrated in *Fig.* 78 *b*), leading to mitral regurgitation. Atrioventricular Canal Defects are common in patients with Down's Syndrome, when there are often only eleven pairs of ribs visible on the chest radiograph (as was the case in this patient although this is not clear from this image). In examinations if you are shown a chest radiograph of a non-cyanosed young child with evidence of heart failure or a large left-to-right shunt be sure to count the ribs, if there are only eleven pairs the child is quite likely to have Down's Syndrome and an Atrioventricular Canal Defect.

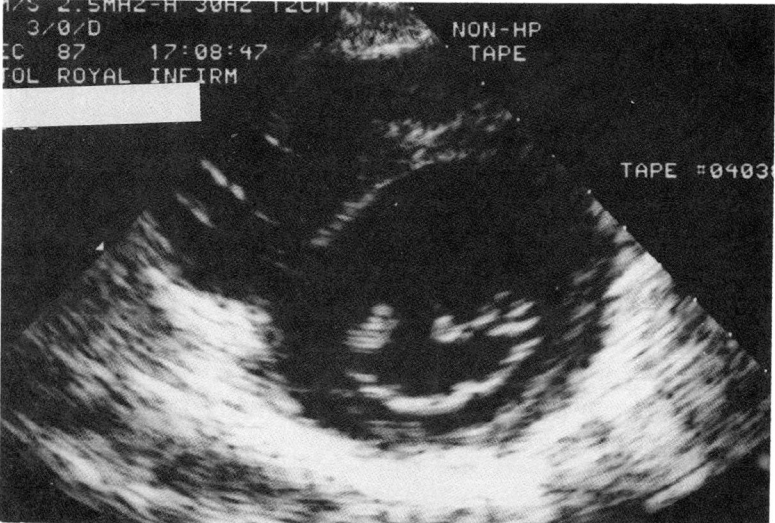

Figure 78 *b*

Case 79

What is this investigation? What abnormalities does it show? What further investigation(s) would you perform? What therapeutic options are available to deal with the main abnormality shown?

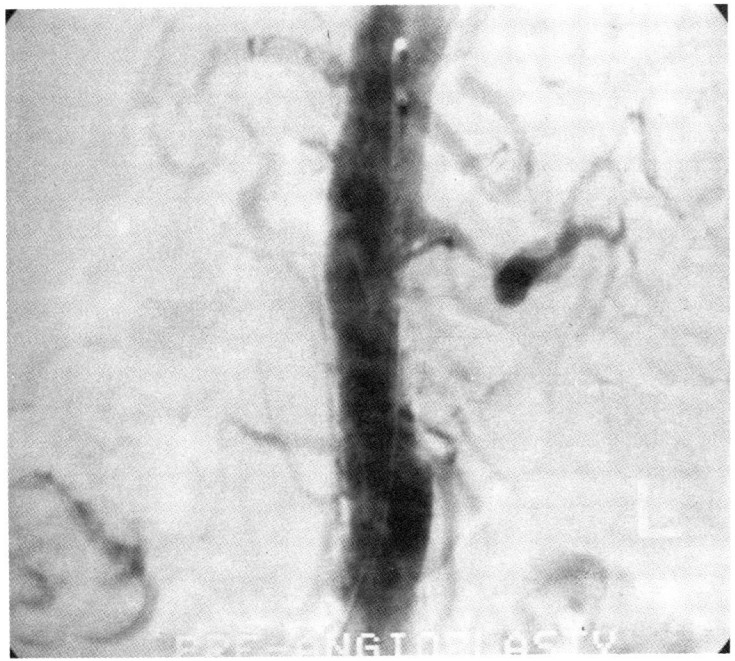

Figure 79a (By courtesy of Professor D. J. Allison)

This is an Intra-arterial Digital Subtraction (DSA) Aortogram which shows that there is Occlusion of the Right Renal Artery and a severe Stenosis of the Left Renal Artery. In addition, although the hepatic and splenic arteries are fairly well opacified there is hardly any opacification of the branches of the superior mesenteric artery (SMA), suggesting that there is a significant Stenosis of the Origin of the SMA. This could be confirmed by a lateral aortogram, which will show stenosis or occlusion of the SMA. There is also a linear subtraction artefact to the right of the lumen of the aorta, which is caused by movement of the calcified aortic wall, indicating that there is extensive disease of the aortic wall.

This patient has a severe renal artery stenosis affecting his only kidney. Although there is debate about the role of other imaging studies (i.e. isotope studies) in selecting patients for renal artery angioplasty, in this situation the patient has a high risk of infarcting his remaining kidney and further imaging of the kidneys is redundant as there is no doubt that the stenosis needs treatment. In this situation angioplasty, with readily available surgical back-up and suitable angioplasty experience, is often the treatment of choice. In this patient the angioplasty was successful in relieving hypertension and improving renal function (*Fig.* 79*b* shows the post-angioplasty angiogram).

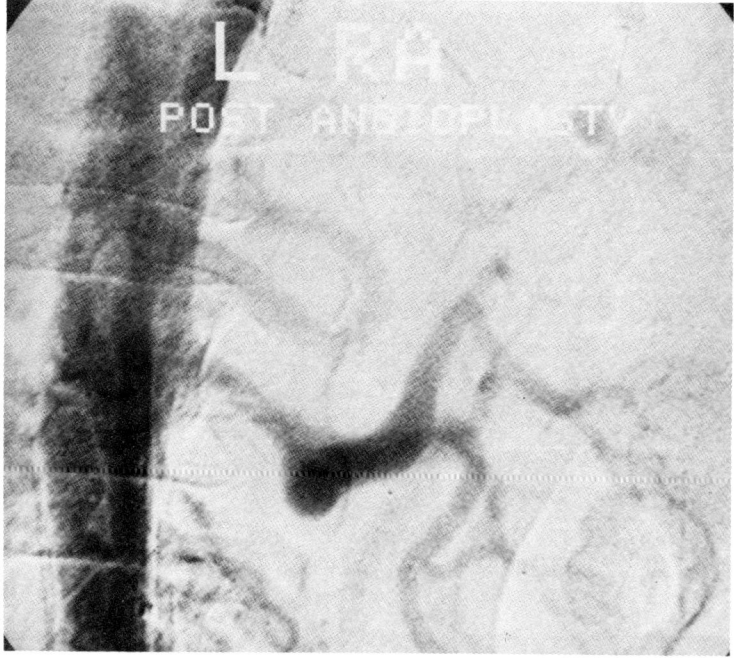

Figure 79*b* (By courtesy of Professor D. J. Allison)

Case 80

What does this chest radiograph of a 7-day-old child show? What are the differential diagnoses? What other imaging techniques are useful in making the diagnosis?

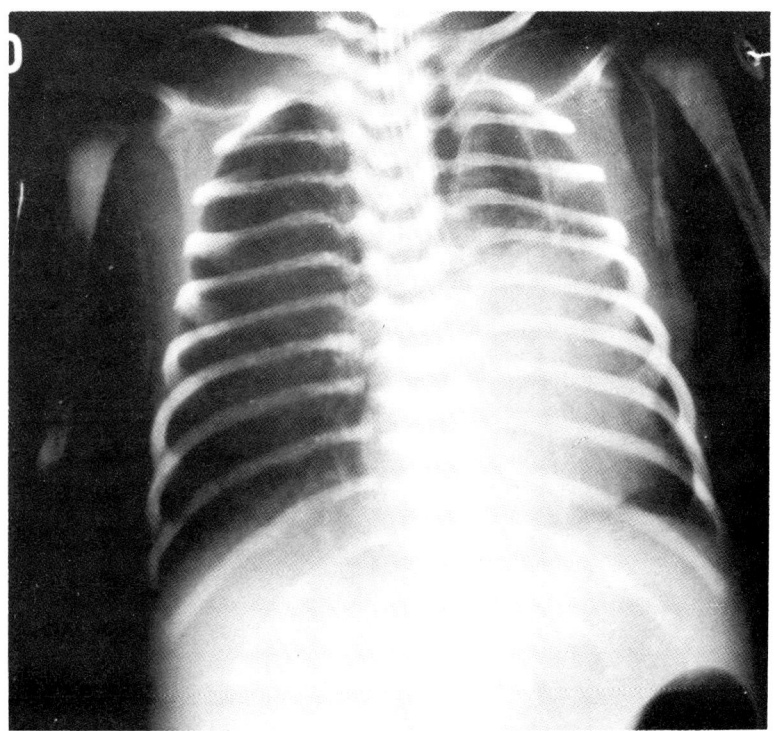

Figure 80a

This chest radiograph shows overinflation of the right lung with depression of the right hemi-diaphragm, shift of the mediastinum to the left and general translucency of the right hemithorax. This indicates that there is Obstruction of the Right Main Bronchus and that the right lung is under Tension. The position of the endotracheal tube in the left main bronchus may seem unsatisfactory but this position was intentional. This position of the endotracheal tube should normally cause underventilation rather than overventilation of the right lung.

The possible causes of this appearance at this age include Foreign Body Inhalation, Bronchial Stenosis, Congenital Lobar Emphysema, Mediastinal Tumours (uncommon) and Vascular Rings. The classic vascular ring anomaly which occludes the right main bronchus is, as was the case in this patient (*Fig.* 80 *b* shows the pulmonary angiogram in this patient), an anomalous left pulmonary artery which passes to the right of the right main bronchus before turning posteriorly and then to the left. This diagnosis is best made by Angiography although in less ill patients a lateral chest radiograph may show a posterior indentation on the trachea. CT Scanning at this age is often difficult to interpret due to the small size of the structures involved but is useful in patients with a suspected mediastinal mass. If the patient has an endotracheal tube this usually produces artefacts which obscure all detail on CT. Other useful techniques include Radiographic Screening, High kVp Radiography (with Magnification) and Bronchography.

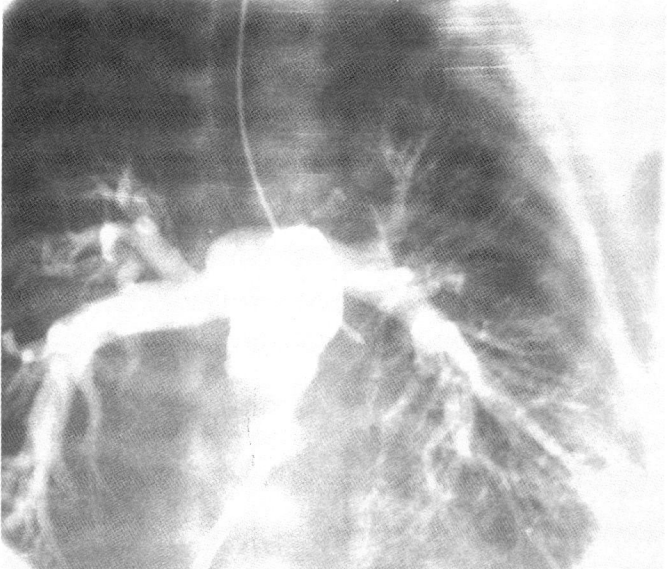

Figure 80 *b*

CARDIOVASCULAR SYSTEM

Bibliography

This list is intentionally short. There are many books and journals which deal with cardiovascular radiology. The references given below are particularly relevant to radiologists in training and others who need to have some knowledge of cardiovascular radiology in their postgraduate examinations.

Essential

Chapman S. and Nakielny R. *Aids to Radiological Differential Diagnosis.* Baillière Tindall, London, 1984. A crucial set of lists of diagnoses for most examinations in which radiographs are discussed.

Either: Grainger R. G. and Allison D. J. (eds) *Diagnostic Radiology: An Anglo-American Textbook of Imaging.* Churchill-Livingstone, London, 1986. Vol. 1, pp. 293–715 and Vol. 3, pp. 1987–2166. For illustrations of most cardiovascular abnormalities likely to be encountered in any examination.

Or: Sutton D. *A Textbook of Radiology* (4th edn). Churchill-Livingstone, London, 1987. Vol. 1, pp. 538–758.

Recommended

Felson B. and Reeder M. M. *Gamuts in Radiology.* Audiovisual Radiology of Cincinnati Inc., Cincinnatti, 1987. For those annoying odd lists and obscure MCQ questions. Do not learn all, or even most of them.

Jefferson K. and Rees R. S. O. *Clinical Cardiac Radiology.* Butterworth, Guildford, 1986. A good explanation of the normal and abnormal plain radiographic features of cardiac disease with very good clinical information.

Simpkins K. Bartlett R. and Parker D. *Radiology Study Guide for Passing the Fellowship.* X-Ray Department, Leeds General Infirmary, Leeds, 1987. This is very much aimed at those who are taking the Fellowship of the Royal College of Radiologists but it contains a lot of sensible and valuable information on how to present oneself in an examination setting. It also contains a large number of up-to-date, if rather long, reading lists for preparing for radiology examinations.

Verel D. and Grainger R. G. *Cardiac Catherization and Angiocardiography* (3rd edn). Churchill-Livingstone, Edinburgh, 1987. For an excellent series of angiograms covering the commoner conditions in congenital and acquired heart disease. Widely available in medical libraries.

Index

Numbers refer to cases

Angiosarcoma 22
Aneurysm
  Aortic 42, 65
  Brachial artery 31
  Popliteal artery 50, 56
  Left ventricle 9
Angioplasty 54, 79
Aortic dissection 1, 21, 34
Aortic stenosis 3, 25, 43, 59
Arteriovenous malformations 22, 39
Arteriovenous fistula 31, 60
Atrial septal defect 26, 55
Atrial thrombus 59

Behçet's disease 11
Blalock shunt 5
Bronchial haemorrhage 64
Bronchogenic cyst 77

Cardiomyopathy 40
Carotid artery stenosis 27, 62
Carotid body tumour 73
Caval thrombosis 61, 68
Cavernosography 71
Coarctation of aorta 10, 17, 36
CT scanning 1, 21, 42, 61
Cyanotic congenital heart disease 5, 18, 49, 58, 69

Digital angiography 11, 16, 27, 36, 41, 43, 60, 65, 71, 73, 79
Doppler 4, 20, 27, 35, 62

Ebstein's anomaly 37
Echocardiography 20, 29, 40, 45, 52, 74
Eisenmenger syndrome 13
Embolisation 22, 39, 64
Empyema 25
Endocardial cushion defect 78
Endocarditis 45, 50

Fallot's Tetralogy 5, 14, 32
Fibrosing mediastinitis 68

Gianturco–Wallace coils 39

Haemosiderosis 4
Hydatid disease 61
Hypertrophic cardiomyopathy 70

Iliac artery occlusion 60

Lung scanning 19

Magnetic resonance imaging 21, 75
Mesocardia 49
Mitral prolapse 74
Mitral regurgitation 35
Mitral stenosis 4, 20, 35, 57, 59
Mitral valvotomy 67

Pacemaker 47, 68
Pectus Excavatum 6
Pericardial constriction 24
Pericardial effusion 29, 44, 75
Persistent ductus arteriosus 33
Pneumopericardium 76
Popliteal artery occlusion 54
Pseudocoarctation 23
Pulmonary artery
  Anomalous origin 80
  Stenosis 6
Pulmonary atresia 5, 14
Pulmonary embolism 19, 28, 46, 51
Pulmonary infarction 28
Pulmonary oedema 8
Pulmonary ossification 57
Pulmonary valve stenosis 2

Renal artery stenosis 79

Single ventricle 18
Subclavian artery, anomalous origin 72
Subclavian steal syndrome 56
Subclavian compression 41

Takayasu's disease 11
Thallium scanning 53
Total anomalous pulmonary venous drainage 7, 48
Transposition of the great arteries 69

Tricuspid atresia 15
Truncus arteriosus 58

Uraemia 8
Uhl's anomaly 14, 37

Valvoplasty 12, 67
Varicocele 30
Vascular rings 72, 80
Venous thrombosis 38
Ventricular septal defect 13, 52